WHAT
LIES
BURIED

Also by Kerry Daynes

The Dark Side of the Mind

WHAT LIES BURIED

A forensic psychologist's true stories of
madness, the bad and the misunderstood

KERRY DAYNES

ENDEAVOUR

First published in Great Britain in 2021 by Endeavour,
an imprint of
Octopus Publishing Group Ltd
Carmelite House
50 Victoria Embankment
London EC4Y 0DZ
www.octopusbooks.co.uk

An Hachette UK Company
www.hachette.co.uk

ISBN 9 781 91306 857 8

A CIP catalogue record for this book is available from the British Library.

Printed and bound in Great Britain

10 9 8 7 6 5 4 3 2 1

This FSC® label means that materials used for the product
have been responsibly sourced.

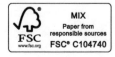

CONTENTS

Prologue 1

1   The Bright Line 19
2   Do No Harm 53
3   In Lies, Truth 87
4   A Frank Confession 123
5   Snap Decisions 161
6   An Empty Room 195
7   Pork and Prejudice 225
8   Out of the Hot Seat 263
9   Blood, Sweat and Fears 301

Epilogue 341
Endnotes 346
Reading Group Questions 355
Author's Acknowledgements 357
About the Author 359

For Dad and Fozzchops

AUTHOR'S NOTE

The stories within these pages are based on my recollections, experience and career as a forensic psychologist. I have taken great care to change all my clients' and colleagues' names, and to disguise locations and other identifying details, in order to protect people's confidentiality, and to keep my bottom firmly on the public benches of the courtroom. After years of seeing people squirm in the dock from up high, I'm not risking my comfy seat for anything.

PROLOGUE

Crime and those who commit it have a habit of dashing our preconceptions.

My working week had been brought to an abrupt halt by an incident involving a kebab skewer and a former arsonist clad in a pinafore and pink rubber gloves. It was an unusual turn of events, to say the least, although probably only in the top ten strange occurrences I'd had to deal with that year.

It was 2011 and I was the weekly contracted psychologist at a forensic step-down project. This is a kind of halfway house, helping people to transition safely from a secure environment to a more independent life. It is an approach that, for the vast majority, proves to be successful. Still, as they say, you can't win 'em all.

The project was set in Laurel House, a large and crumbling Edwardian mansion which stood on a main artery into a busy northern city, hidden from view by a screen of glossy-leafed hedges. Most of those driving past would have no idea what, or perhaps more importantly who, was inside. Had they looked more closely they would have seen that the sash windows had been specially adapted so they only opened up to a maximum of four inches and that the front door, with its once-magnificent stained-glass panels, was only accessible with a magnetic fob key.

My job was to carry out psychological assessments and

therapies with the residents – all male and all ex-offenders who, it was hoped, would eventually go on to live crime-free, independent lives. These were not your petty criminals. Their convictions ranged from murder and violent assault to sexual offences and arson. Most had come from medium- and low-secure psychiatric hospitals, facilities built in the 1980s and 90s to bridge the gap between high-secure hospitals like Broadmoor, Ashworth and Rampton, and community psychiatric services, though some had been released from prisons. What they shared was a high risk of reoffending.

They were all considered 'mentally disordered offenders', meaning they'd been diagnosed with a 'disorder or disability of the mind' that was believed to have played a role in their criminal behaviour or they had gone on to develop one after their conviction. For some, this meant severe mood difficulties or distress that manifested itself in visions, voices or strange beliefs. For others, it meant they had learning difficulties or neurological conditions, like autism.

Personally, I always recoil when I hear the term 'mentally disordered' (whether or not it is applied to those with a criminal record). It sounds so mechanical, like a person is a defunct vending machine where the crisps keep getting stuck and an 'out of order' sign is taped to the glass. I don't think of my clients as broken bits of apparatus with a metaphorical screw loose. They are people. People with differences, people with problems.

My job was to work out what these problems were, where they came from and, most importantly, what could be done to keep the ex-offenders on the right track. I worked closely with the local Multi-Agency Public Protection Arrangements (MAPPA) panel, a forum run by police and probation to supervise potentially dangerous individuals.

Which brings me to the incident with the kebab skewer. Despite the eclectic list of houseguests, each with a unique and testing set of issues, the hours leading up to 'kebabgate' had been unremarkable. Perhaps others wouldn't see it that way, given that questions like 'Have the voices felt any less powerful this week?' and 'How have you been getting on with keeping your masturbation diary?' are not your average water-cooler chit-chat. But in a place like this, it's par for the course. That's not to say I'm desensitized or blasé about my clients: far from it. In fact, the more time I've spent doing this work and the more people I meet, the more curious I become about the human experience.

I am often asked what attracted me to forensic psychology; why I was drawn to spending my days with people whom society has judged to be beyond the pale. My stock response is to say I wanted to help people and contribute to a world with fewer victims in it. And that would be true. But it sounds suspiciously like something a beauty-pageant contestant might say, followed by 'and to achieve world peace'.

A more complete and (possibly) enlightening answer is that ever since I was a child I've been attracted to the darker side of life. The macabre, strange and unorthodox happenings and seemingly inexplicable twists and turns in a plot have always been irresistible to me.

I loved Roald Dahl's *Tales of the Unexpected*. The unforgettable theme tune was swirling and creepily dream-like, as if it belonged in the haunted house of a crumbling fairground, perhaps drifting from a cobwebbed music box with a wind-up, twirling ballerina on top. I'd watch the silhouetted girl dancing in front of the flames in the opening titles while holding onto a cushion I could hide behind as the story unfolded. Even if I'd known then that the dancer was actually a secretary from Berkshire, roped in by her boyfriend whose job it was to create the titles, it wouldn't have dented my willingness to suspend my disbelief. I found the tales as grippingly intriguing as they were disquieting.

I also read the short stories the episodes were based on. My favourite was *The Landlady*: a young man arrives at a guesthouse and when he reads the guest book it begins to dawn on him that all the names are of young men who have gone missing. And then the landlady reveals a passion for taxidermy ...

In the TV introduction to *The Landlady*, Roald Dahl says, 'If any of you are tempted to think it's all pretty far-fetched, then you should stop and think and ask yourself seriously whether such a thing as this could really happen? The answer is yes, of course it could.' And he was right. It has been suggested that one of Dahl's tales, *Lamb to the Slaughter*, inspired Anthony Hardy's choice of weapon when he attacked his wife in 1982 (he used a frozen bottle of water, rather than an un-defrosted leg of lamb). The serial killer from Camden was later handed a whole life sentence in 2003 for the murder and dismemberment of three women.

My childish fascination with the shady corners of life, the hairpin bends in the stories I read and the dark dead ends in true-crime accounts drew me into a world I didn't want to leave. As I grew older, the interest became less voyeuristic and evolved into a much deeper, intellectual curiosity about the psychological complexities of people.

On the day of kebabgate, I'd finished my shift at 5pm and, hoping to avoid sitting in nose-to-tail traffic on the M60 back home to Manchester, I'd stayed behind to have dinner with the staff and residents. This may not sound like the most enjoyable early-evening plan but the food was free and edible, one of the few perks of the job. Chicken and vegetable kebabs were on the menu that day, which I'd enjoyed before. As always, the food had been prepared by the part-time chef in a locked kitchen (a sensible precaution, so the residents didn't have easy access to sharp knives or cooking utensils).

The drill was that when you'd finished your meal in the dining room, you carried your plate and cutlery to a separate galley kitchen across the corridor. The residents took it in turns to wash up. Nigel was doing the dishes that evening. A shy and uncommunicative man in his early thirties, Nigel had a mild learning disability and I couldn't help but notice that he had some of the tell-tale signs of foetal alcohol syndrome: he was unusually small in stature, had a thin upper lip, a wide space between his eyes, and his philtrum (the area between the top lip and the nose) was completely flat. He had been at the project for about four months. I'd seen him around but had hardly spoken to him during that time, though I knew he was suspected of using drugs.

When I'd polished off my only slightly rubbery chicken, I walked into the galley kitchen and set my dirty plate and cutlery down beside the sink, saying thank you to Nigel as I did so. He was alone, standing at one of the two stainless-steel sinks on the left-hand side of the narrow room, wearing a pair of pink Marigolds and a blue-striped apron and staring at the pyramid of dishes and soapsuds in front of him.

I was about to turn and leave when, completely unexpectedly, Nigel ran straight at me.

'Huuuuh!' A weird, animal-like sound rebounded around the stark kitchen. It took me a moment to realize the unfamiliar noise had come from me, and then another second to register that I'd made that sound because Nigel had punched me in the stomach. The blow seemed to have forced the air out of my body, as if I were a punchbag that had had some stuffing knocked out of it.

'You've killed me!' Nigel exclaimed.

I remember taking a second to appreciate what a classic textbook example of projection that was, given that what Nigel really meant was, 'I think I've killed you.' A pretty useless first thought, I admit, given that textbooks aren't that much use when you've just been whacked in the stomach.

'No one is dead,' I said quietly, my hand automatically reaching for where he'd struck me, just below my ribs. 'Nobody has died.'

That's when the realization struck me. Nigel hadn't

punched me at all. There was a long thin metal rod sticking out of my body. He had stabbed me with a chicken kebab skewer. The unlikely weapon was lodged firmly in my stomach, protruding at a right angle to my abdomen.

I can remember feeling sickened by how easily my body had been punctured. Only about six inches of the ten-inch skewer were still visible and you didn't need to be a maths genius to work out I had a full four inches of metal lodged inside my stomach. It had gone straight through the soft skin beneath my sternum, as if I were a piece of halloumi.

Nigel looked panic-stricken and desperate to escape. He was dancing from side to side like a hummingbird in mating season, eyes flicking towards the door behind me, his head twitching wildly.

'I think you should go to your room now, please,' I said firmly. I was on autopilot and sounded rather schoolmarmish, which is a typical, involuntary reaction of mine in a difficult situation. I'm trained not to panic and my instinct at work is to try to channel what I hope, at least, is a reassuring air of calm authority, even when I have a stick run through me like I'm a piece of 1980s party food.

I backed out of the narrow kitchen as Nigel scurried off. The alternative would have been to sound the safety alarm on my belt but I made a split-second decision that this might have put me in more danger. I didn't want other people cramming into this confined space, trapping me with a spooked Nigel and a sink full of kebab skewers.

As soon as Nigel had gone, I walked the few feet to the

staff office and banged on the locked door with the palm of my hand.

Laura, a young and fairly new support worker, employed to supervise and assist the residents, opened the door. She gasped in disbelief at the sight of me impaled on a metal spike. To be fair, I must have been a sight to behold. My breathing was getting increasingly rapid and a red circle of blood was seeping into my white blouse, which meant my mid-section was beginning to resemble a Japanese flag in a strong breeze.

'Shall I pull it out?' Laura said.

There is always one person on duty per shift who is trained in first aid; I was guessing it wasn't her.

'No!' I growled, spitting out something incomprehensible about not even *thinking* about touching me or the skewer. I'd gone from head-teacher mode to sounding like the possessed girl in *The Exorcist.* Somehow, I managed not to swear, which I thought was superbly professional of me, given the circumstances. 'Call an ambulance!' I ordered.

Laura grabbed the phone and started frantically dialling 999. After three failed attempts, I snatched the receiver off her, punched in '9' to get an outside line, then dialled 999 myself and shoved the handset back at her. *I'll apologize to her later*, I thought.

The paramedics arrived within about ten minutes. By that time, two members of staff were guarding Nigel, who had fled to his bedroom on the floor above. Meanwhile, I was being looked after by the unit manager, a dead ringer for

Basil Fawlty who was trying, awkwardly, to distract me with some light conversation. He wasn't getting very far. I was in shock and deteriorating. All I could think about was whether Nigel had washed the skewer before he stabbed me with it or if it still had bits of chicken carcass clinging to it.

'It must have been a completely random attack,' Basil said, changing tack.

I gritted my teeth and grunted. There is no such thing as an entirely random assault. The assailant has to either wait for an ideal opportunity or create one. Plenty of other people had been in and out of the kitchen but I was one of the very few women in the building that day. Not only that, I was the least familiar to Nigel and, at five foot three, probably the smallest.

'So don't blame yourself,' Basil went on. I shot him the most withering look I could muster and he patted my arm.

We were both relieved when the paramedics arrived. They steered me expertly into the ambulance and drove off, blue light flashing, as I wondered how I was going to explain this to my parents and if my insides would ever function properly again.

I had a minor operation to remove the offending piece of metal and was kept in hospital overnight. Fortunately, Nigel had managed to avoid doing serious damage; the skewer had only punctured the top of my stomach, despite leaving me with a two-inch scar.

In this line of work, when you manage to escape with your life, a rite of passage on the road to recovery is being mercilessly teased by your colleagues. When I went back to work the following week, the staff at the project started to call me Donna. 'Shish, that's a really bad joke,' I responded, pointing out that it's actually a shish kebab that involves a skewer and not a doner. They carried on regardless. Accuracy never gets in the way of a good piss-taking.

At least I could dine out on the drama. A few days after leaving hospital, I was due to meet some friends for afternoon tea and was looking forward to regaling them with the tale. It was guaranteed to be a show-stopper, wasn't it?

'What's new with you, Kerry?'

There it was. My cue to tell the story that would surely trump all others round the table that day.

'Well . . .' I said, leaving a theatrical pause.

All eyes were on me. *Is it still schadenfreude if you revel in your own misfortune?* I wondered.

'What? Go on.'

'I got stabbed in the stomach at work!'

I delivered my shocking news with a wide-eyed flourish, deliberately leaving out the fact that the weapon used against me had been a kebab skewer.

I waited for the stunned gasps and barrage of questions about how something like this could have happened to me in my place of work. I continued to wait.

Not one of my friends looked in the least bit surprised. My words rolled like tumbleweed across the teacups and cream cakes, as my friends shrugged and raised their eyebrows.

'Weren't you wearing a stab-proof vest? Surely you have to wear one of those, don't you?'

'What?' I stuttered 'No! Why would I wear a stab-proof vest? I'm hardly in the riot police, am I?'

One of my girlfriends pointed out that I worked with a load of 'nutters' and so, obviously, I needed to protect myself by dressing head-to-toe in Kevlar.

Her reaction surprised me. How could any of my educated and usually tolerant friends have such a biased and discriminatory view of the people I worked with? They knew nothing about them, apart from the fact they had mental-health struggles and had broken the law.[1]

'I do *not* need to wear a stab-proof vest to work,' I insisted, gobsmacked. 'This is not a normal everyday occurrence. This was A. Very. Bad. Day.'

I could tell no one was convinced.

Part of the reason for my friends' ignorance is that the people I work with live out of sight and out of mind in institutions that we know little about. They occupy a blind spot in our collective consciousness. Although we are constantly drip-fed information about the people who commit crime through click-bait headlines, one-dimensional news reports and 'expert' soundbites, we don't truly engage with them. We write them off as irredeemable, then move on to the next ramped-up and dumbed-down news story.

My friends certainly weren't the first to make this mistake. Myths and stigma surrounding mental-health problems, and

---

1 And they wouldn't be hearing anything from me that day about the man I've called 'Nigel' here or any other patient – confidentiality is a core principle of my profession. Gossiping about my clients is a strict no-no.

in particular their perceived link to indiscriminate violence, have persisted throughout history.

For centuries, people who committed a crime were viewed as sinners and punished by imprisonment, torture and execution (or perhaps all three), regardless of their motivations or mental state. It wasn't until the 19th century, when psychiatry and criminology began to develop as two distinct but interrelated disciplines, that people started to closely consider the mental state of people who broke the law. The case of James Hadfield, who tried to assassinate George III at the Theatre Royal in 1800 by shooting at him during the national anthem, moved things on apace. Supported by one of the leading barristers of the era, Hadfield was able to successfully argue that his actions were the direct result of irrational beliefs, linked to head injuries sustained when he had fought against the French a few years earlier.

The judge faced a problem. He was clear in his mind that Hadfield's act was the result of 'insanity' and therefore he should not be convicted of the offence but also that he could not be allowed to walk free and potentially reoffend. The solution was for Parliament to speedily pass the Criminal Lunatics Act and ship Hadfield to Bethlem (the psychiatric hospital more commonly known as Bedlam). It was a ground-breaking judgement, setting in stone the distinction between 'mad' and 'bad' that in many ways has continued to the present day.

Hadfield spent the rest of his life in Bedlam. It was not a place where anyone would want to go; it was a squalid institution where, until 1760, members of the public had been allowed to come to gawp at the inmates, as if they were freaks in a circus. The hospital became enduringly synonymous in popular culture with dangerous, scary derangement, inspiring several horror books, films and TV series, most notably *Bedlam*, a 1946 film starring Boris Karloff. The stigma of being mentally distressed stuck like feathers on tar, the myths perpetuating down the years and lodging in the public's perception of all people suffering with mental-health problems, whether or not they had committed crimes or were a danger to the public.

Until only a few generations ago, psychiatrists were known as 'alienists', reflecting the belief that they were dealing with people who almost belonged to a different species. Some doctors lived up to the description more than others. Dr James Prichard, influential author of the 1835 'Treatise on Insanity and Other Disorders Affecting the Mind', performed autopsies on his patients, concluding that brain 'disease' and other physical abnormalities contributed to a special kind of madness that rendered sufferers morally bankrupt and prone to committing 'every species of mischief'. He called for such 'dangerous lunatics', rather than being punished for their misdemeanours, to instead be secluded from society and given 'treatments' such as bloodletting, surprise ice baths, emetics to encourage vomiting and, his particular favourite, being spun round in a rotary machine in the hope that their 'moral insanity' would be, quite literally, shaken out of them.

Fast-forward to today and it doesn't take a thorough reading of tabloid headlines to find the modern equivalent of Prichard's dehumanizing language and ideas. For 'dangerous lunatics' we now read 'psycho' or 'crazed killers'. Psychiatry may have moved on somewhat with the times but stigma and cliché have clung on like leeches in a phlebotomy, keeping alive myths that should have been abandoned along with the 'insanity-shaker' machine.

Let's be clear: the reality is that talk of so-called 'axe-wielding schizos', 'murderous psychos' and 'evil monsters' who carry out 'twisted attacks' are largely inaccurate, exaggerated caricatures, manufactured and spun by the media and the entertainment industry. The unfortunate and very unhelpful consequence of this is that the public overestimates the risk posed by people with mental-health issues, viewing them as more violent and more dangerous than the data suggests. What we should emphasize is the fact that not all 'mentally disordered' people are dangerous (and not all dangerous people are 'mentally disordered').

When you work at the more turbulent end of psychology as I do, you quickly learn that when violence does happen, there is always more to it than meets the eye. My job would be simple (and boring) if I could pull a label out of my diagnostic tombola, stick it on my client's head and claim that as an all-encompassing explanation for their actions. It is never that simple because there is always a more complex story hidden beneath the surface.

Having deduced that Nigel had chosen me as his victim

because I was the easiest target, my focus turned to what made him choose a victim – any victim – in the first place.

His file told me he'd spent a large part of his childhood in care. When he was ten years old, he set a fire in his foster-carer's bedroom, egged on by other boys. At 17, he moved into shared accommodation as a stepping-stone to independent living. After ten days, he piled all his clothes on top of a mattress, lit a fire and, after watching it take hold, walked to a phone box and dialled 999. This ensured that his next home was a young offenders' institution, where he spent nearly four years. The following attempt at living independently ended when he made a hoax bomb call to police after setting fire to a bin he had stuffed full of rubbish inside a bus station. Nigel was subsequently convicted of a second arson and detained under the Mental Health Act in a locked psychiatric hospital. He stayed there for seven years and had just completed a group Arson Awareness Programme prior to his move to the step-down project.

People set deliberate fires for a number of reasons, including insurance fraud, covering up a crime, revenge, making a political or social statement or even for sexual excitement. It's common for those who commit arson to have problems communicating and expressing themselves. Some lack the ability to prevent themselves from being overwhelmed by emotions and have poor problem-solving skills. They see setting fire to something as their 'last viable option' – the only possible way to escape a situation they no longer want to be in.

This described Nigel: his fire-starting aligned with periods in his life when he felt trapped and miserable, with no other way of effecting the change he wanted.

I discovered, some time later, that a couple of local men who used the same probation office as Nigel had confessed to using him as their 'spice pig', meaning they were forcing him to take concoctions of synthetic drugs in order to test their safety before they sold them on the street. This is not uncommon: people with learning disabilities are often preyed upon by unscrupulous drug dealers.

So, given his circumstances, skewering me was a rational, though ill-advised, action. It may not sound rational, but Nigel was desperate to move away from the dealers living near the step-down facility and experience had taught him that breaking the law was a ticket to 'somewhere else'. He had shifted from addressing his dilemma with a lighted match to assault with a sharp object but the function of the behaviour was the same.

After attacking me, he got his wish and was transferred to a medium-secure hospital. I wondered if he would spend the next seven years completing a different out-of-the-box programme – Skewer Awareness, perhaps? – or if this time he would receive the help he needed to develop some altogether more practical communication and problem-solving skills.

I am unlikely to ever forget Nigel, particularly when I look down and see the scar on my stomach. But in a perverse way, it serves as a useful reminder not to jump to conclusions about the people in my care. After all, each of us has a unique tale to tell and a backstory that explains a great deal about who we are and why we behave the way we do. I see people – all people – like the living, breathing pages of a book, the plots of our lives shaped by our place and time in the world, the relationships we foster and the influences and events we are exposed to, and respond to, on our life's journey.

The people you are about to read of here, whether they are confessed killers, frightened and frightening hospital patients or victims, are all walking storybooks, just like the rest of us. Multi-layered characters with chapters already written, plot twists to navigate and a narrative that is yet to reach its conclusion. My hope in writing about them is to give some compassion and humanity back to those who are often denied both.

Perhaps if we listen more and judge less then we'll see that there may be a little bit of their story in all of us.

CHAPTER ONE
THE BRIGHT LINE

'We need this argument resolved and we know you don't sit on the fence, Kerry. Is the defendant lying about hearing voices or not?'

Mad or bad? That's what the prosecution lawyer wanted to know. It's the perennial question that lies at the heart of forensic psychology, embedded in the minds of the press and public as much as it is in law and policy. A criminal must surely be one or the other.

This was a high-profile homicide case and my opinion might make the difference between a killer serving a mandatory life sentence (with a minimum 'tariff' of years they must spend in prison before being eligible for parole), a shorter prison sentence or, more likely, being detained indefinitely under the Mental Health Act in a secure hospital. Once again, as I had so many times before, I was being asked to put a definitive label on a person, one that had the potential to change the course of his life. I was reminded of that scene in the classic film adaptation *Willy Wonka & the Chocolate Factory*, when Gene Wilder explains how his Eggdicator machine determines the difference between a good egg and a bad egg: 'If it's a good egg it's shined up and shipped out all over the world. But if it's a bad egg...down the chute.'

As a child, I loved watching Veruca Salt disappearing down the garbage hatch after threatening to scream if she didn't get all the outlandish treats and presents she demanded. All it took was for her to stand on the Eggdicator machine and her fate was sealed, just like that. The arrow swiftly pointed to 'bad' and she was suitably dispatched. There wasn't a shred of doubt in my mind that the spoiled, obnoxious little girl had got her just deserts.

Real life isn't so straightforward, though there are plenty of lawyers and other professionals who behave as if it could be.

'Kerry, what's wrong with this one?'

'She is in a state of intense distress because…'

'Yes, but what's *wrong* with her?'

'Well, she meets diagnostic criteria for schizoaffective disorder as a result of…'

Slap! A 'mad' sticker is plonked on the person's forehead before you can blink. Clunk! The lever's pulled and she plummets through the hatch marked 'psychiatric hospital'.

'Wait! I wanted to tell you…'

'Sorry, can't stop, the production line is busy today. Next! What's wrong with this one?'

'Um, he doesn't have any significant mental-health difficulties at the moment but…'

Slap! The 'bad' label is whacked on and you watch in frustration as he hurtles at breakneck speed down the fast-track chute to prison.

I often look around prison wings, hospital wards and courtrooms in despair. I'm dealing with multi-faceted human beings. People with nuanced stories and incredibly complex issues.

My client, the next to be processed through our legal system, was Michael. At the age of 17, he had killed one man and tried to stab another to death. He had pleaded not guilty to murder and attempted murder but guilty to the lesser crimes of manslaughter and attempted manslaughter on the grounds of diminished responsibility. The issue for the Crown Prosecution Service (CPS) was whether or not they would accept his plea. If they did, he could be sentenced without the need for a lengthy trial.

Diminished responsibility is only a *partial* defence to murder and doesn't allow anyone to wriggle completely off the hook. It was introduced into English law in 1957 to acknowledge that a substantial grey area exists between 'sanity' and 'insanity'. Whereas someone claiming insanity at the time of committing a crime must prove that they were fully incapable of distinguishing right from wrong (a tough position for even those in the most dire of mental states to successfully argue), a person claiming diminished responsibility must only show that he or she was suffering from an 'abnormality of mind' which 'substantially impaired' their level of responsibility.

The concept of diminished responsibility is a helpful one, designed to encourage a thorough exploration of all the information and circumstances in a case and stop the jury becoming bogged down in, or beguiled by, any one source of evidence. This includes opinions on the defendant's state of mind provided by psychiatrists and psychologists like me. That's the theory, anyway. In practice, this antiquated legal machine has a habit of backfiring.

Four psychiatrists, instructed by Michael's defence team, had assessed him over varying lengths of time. They concluded that, at the time of the attacks, he had been acting upon delusional beliefs and suffering auditory hallucinations (psychiatry-speak for hearing voices) compelling him to kill. Two of the experts had given him a diagnosis of schizophrenia, one had opted for brief psychotic disorder and the fourth, just for variety, had thrown schizoaffective disorder into the mix. All four experts were convinced that Michael was not entirely culpable for his actions and, ideally, should be dropped through the chute marked 'psychiatric hospital'.

However, a fifth psychiatrist, instructed by the Crown, did not agree. The well-respected Dr Bradling, known for his Savile Row suits and loud bow ties, was of the firm opinion that Michael had hoodwinked his colleagues. The boy had an 'emerging psychopathic personality disorder', he said. In his view, Michael would inevitably become a full-blown psychopath as he matured. Yet despite hardly giving the teenager a spotless bill of mental health, Dr Bradling argued that Michael's emerging psychopathic personality did not 'substantially impair' his criminal responsibility.

Personality, unlike psychosis, is not something you 'have' or experience. It is who you are. Diagnosing someone with a 'personality disorder' is a bit like declaring them to be a loaded gun. The insidious implication here is that the person possesses a particularly unusual and virulent strain of nastiness that might be triggered at any time. Nevertheless, those diagnosed with a personality disorder are obliged to keep their supposed proclivities in check, which is not the most reasonable expectation when you think about it. It's a bit like owning a pet scorpion and being outraged when it stings you. No wonder critics describe it as more of a 'pejorative judgement' than a clinical diagnosis.

Michael was abnormally aggressive, scheming, callous and a liar to boot, Dr Bradling concluded, and should be punished accordingly with a prison sentence.

It is not unusual for opinions regarding a defendant's mental state to be fiercely contested. I've spent more hours than I care to count in courtrooms being grilled on the finer points of someone else's inner mental workings, when another professional with very similar training to mine has come up with markedly different interpretations. Although the overriding duty of an expert witness is to provide an independent, unbiased opinion, the cynic in me sometimes muses that it's curious how often views differ according to which side is paying the expert's bill.

The difference between a forensic psychologist and a psychiatrist is that psychiatrists are medically trained and, as such, they are medics first and forensic specialists second. Psychologists are not medically qualified, although we go through a rigorous period of at least six years' training to reach chartered and/or registered status, the quality marks of a true psychology professional. Psychologists cannot prescribe medication but we are trained in talking therapies and have a range of questionnaires, standardized tests, interview templates and psychological theories at our disposal. The CPS had brought me in to offer a fresh perspective and play referee between the eminent doctors. As I started trawling through the eight-inch-thick pile of witness statements and transcripts of Michael's police interviews (all with accompanying videos) I tried to wipe my mind clean of anybody else's thinking.

Michael was barely an adult, having only recently turned 18. When I looked at his photograph, he reminded me of Harry Potter's friend Ron Weasley, before his voice broke and he grew stubble. The media machine had already gone into overdrive, predictably casting him as the 'baby-faced killer'. This was not an assessment I was taking on lightly.

According to his mother, Michael had been an active and adventurous child. In 2003, at the age of 16, he'd passed a tough Royal Navy recruitment process and achieved his ambition of joining the Marines. He stayed for just 18 months. She'd never quite got to the bottom of what caused him to suddenly leave.

In August 2005, Michael killed Finbar Jackson, a 32-year-old homeless man who had been released from a short prison sentence three months earlier. Finbar had left prison in the clothes he stood up in and with a discharge grant of a few pounds, his discharge papers and a travel card.

He began sleeping rough, joining the ranks of the 30 per

cent of homeless people who were once behind bars. On the night of his death, Finbar had been drinking heavily, found his way to the entrance of a park and slumped down on the grass. At 12.30am, a young man spoke to him, asking, 'Are you alright, mate?' When Finbar responded with a slurred 'yes' he gave him the remains of a packet of chips.

Four and a half hours later, Michael snuck out of his house, via the kitchen window. His mum and stepfather were asleep in bed and he didn't want to disturb them by opening the front door. He readily admitted this to the police and also told them that he was looking for someone to kill that morning. He went equipped with a large kitchen knife and wore thin grey driving gloves so as to avoid leaving any fingerprints.

He turned left out of his house towards a park a mile and a half away. When he came across Finbar he was lying in a foetal position, snoring softly and smelling strongly of alcohol. Michael mimed for the interviewing officers how he had knelt over his victim, rolled him over and jabbed him in the chest with the knife. Finbar let out a shriek and then Michael slit his throat three times, completely severing the soft tissues at the front of his neck. The cuts were so deep the blade went through to Finbar's vertebral column. Michael then cut a length of material from the wadded lining of the dying man's coat, forced it into his mouth and, as far as he could, down what remained of his throat.

Michael took the knife home, ran it under the tap until the water turned clear and the next day he buried it down a rabbit hole. He put his bloodstained T-shirt, gloves, jacket and blood-splattered trainers into a plastic bag and left it in a neighbour's black bin to be collected with the rubbish. Finbar's body was found by a dog walker at 7.30am the same day.

It's an uncomfortable truth that not all deceased people are viewed equally in the eyes of the media. Victims exist in a strict hierarchy of newsworthiness, according to their perceived virtue, the role they (supposedly) played in their own demise and how they score on the barometer of public opinion that crudely assesses the value and potential of a life lost. If a person merits that clichéd old chestnut, 'he/she had the world at their feet', then their death is likely to be far more widely reported. A classic example is Rachel Nickell, the blonde, beautiful and devoted young mother who was killed while out walking with her two-year-old son on Wimbledon Common in 1992. The tabloid papers' ideal of a victim. Her death sparked such intense public furore and media scrutiny that her son and his father fled the country to escape it.

The violent nature of Finbar's demise was shocking but despite – or perhaps because of – the sad circumstances he was in, his story did not attract much attention beyond the local press. The (so far) fruitless police investigation was soon forgotten. Michael may well have got away with killing Finbar had he stopped there, but he didn't.

Three months later, Michael attempted to kill 51-year-old newsagent Syed Akbar, a popular, hard-working member of the community who was described as having a 'smile for everyone'. This time, the attack resonated with the public, sparking extensive press coverage and a tidal wave of anxiety.

The attack on Syed had come in the wake of the 7/7 bombings in London, when concern about the rise in retaliatory hate crimes against the Muslim population was running high. The newspapers instantly began speculating about whether the attack had been racially or religiously motivated. 'Gentle family man targeted for wearing a kufi skullcap' the headlines declared, while praising the 'popular local figure' who 'fought for his life in frenzied racist attack'. People were not only appalled, they were frightened.

It's interesting how fear can simultaneously mobilize and paralyse a community. Women started to walk in pairs and police handed out thousands of personal-attack alarms to local residents. First in line were those in ethnic-minority groups who felt exposed and vulnerable. Still, the measures were not enough to stop the once vibrant community shrinking in terror, the streets becoming almost empty after dark.

In January 2006, approximately two months after the attack on Syed, the hyper-vigilance of one local resident paid off. Susan Cunliffe, a bakery worker driving home from a night shift, spotted Michael as he wandered the streets in the early hours of the morning. Something didn't feel right to her. She listened to her gut instinct and phoned the police. The two officers who responded found Michael with a hammer and a long-bladed knife in his pockets. When they asked him what he was doing he volunteered nonchalantly, 'I'm looking for someone to kill.' He added, 'It's the voices...they want me to make a sacrifice.'

*

The maximum-security hospital Michael was sent to for assessment after his arrest had been built in the 1860s and looked firmly stuck in that era. The Victorian architecture appeared fairly impressive from the outside, with its series of T-shaped red-brick buildings and their narrow panelled windows, not to mention the imposing clock tower at the entrance. It was a different story once you stepped behind the façade: everything on the inside was shabby, dingy and grim. In just a couple of years, the hospital would be declared unfit for purpose and undergo a much-needed rebuild, the soulless wards with their flaking paint and blind corners replaced with light, airy, practical spaces decorated in calming pastel shades.

It takes a long time to enter any secure hospital, let alone a maximum-security one. As usual, I had all my belongings, bar a pen and papers, taken off me and placed in a locker on arrival. I waited in the air lock, the space between two oppositely opening and closing electronic doors, before being directed through airport-style searches, X-ray and metal-detection portals and photo-identification points. I was then sniffed over by an enthusiastic drug-detection dog and only then, 40 minutes after I'd arrived, could I embark on the long open-air walk across the sprawling internal grounds to the unit where I was meeting Michael.

I'd been in this hospital many times before but its setting always affected me. It is remote, hence the prison euphemism 'being sent to cottage country'. There's a large white statue of an angel and a small cemetery, where some of the asylum superintendents from when the place was first built are buried alongside the unmarked graves of patients who died during their detention and had no family to take them. No escape for them, even in death.

The statue always reminds me of those creepy weeping angels that featured in a few episodes of *Dr Who*. Every time I pass it, I feel compelled to turn back around and look at it again just in case it has crept up behind me while my back was turned.

I was relieved when I eventually arrived at the 12-bed admission block and heard the click of the door lock behind me. I was steered into a cell-like room housing a table, three chairs and one large spider who was attached to the light-fitting, packing an unfortunate fly into a gossamer suitcase. A nurse popped his head around the door and explained that they didn't have enough personal alarms to go round the staff today, let alone visitors. He pointed to a green alarm button on the wall that I could use if I needed to call for help. 'But I don't think you'll get much trouble from this one,' he added. 'I'll go and get him for you.'

I sat and waited, wondering about the person I was about to meet. Statistically speaking, the chances of being killed by a stranger who is in the midst of psychosis is about the same as being struck by lightning – one in ten million. Around 50 homicides per year, or 10 per cent of all UK homicides, are committed by those with severe mental-health problems. Every one of those cases is devastating for those involved and their families; nevertheless, it means that the proportion of people diagnosed with severe mental-health problems who go on to kill is tiny.

Michael's confession to his attack on Syed had been as dry and matter-of-fact as his description of Finbar's last moments. Once again, he had left his home at 5am, via the kitchen window. He told the police that he was wearing knitted gloves and carrying a Swiss army knife. This time he turned right, heading to a housing estate on the edge of a common about a mile away. He wandered around for an hour, he said, and Syed was the first person he saw.

The newsagent had got up at 5.30am, organized the papers for delivery and was sweeping up outside his shop. Michael watched him go in and out of the doorway for five or six minutes before running up behind him, grabbing him by the face with his left hand and putting his right arm over and across his shoulders, to cut his neck. Michael told police that he'd adjusted his technique this time, hoping to avoid being covered in blood as he had been when he'd killed Finbar.

Things didn't go to plan. Syed's body went limp with fear before Michael could slit his throat. The pair lost their balance and fell to the floor. An undignified struggle broke out, during which Michael stabbed Syed twice in the neck, narrowly missing his jugular vein. The knife caught Syed superficially in the chest and head, and cut his hands as he tried to defend himself. He rolled over just as Michael lunged at him again. The knife missed its target and broke as it struck the pavement. Michael explained how he then forced his hand down Syed's throat, grabbing at his tongue.

Lights suddenly flicked on upstairs and at a house across the street and Michael took this as his cue to bolt, leaving Syed to be found by his horrified wife and daughter. They called the emergency services, who got there just in time to save his life. Meanwhile, Michael went home and washed his clothes. A week later, he left them outside a charity shop along with some bric-a-brac, the final details divulged to the police as bluntly and impassively as the rest.

My task was to evaluate Michael's mental state at the 'material time' – i.e., the time of his offences. But months had passed since the attack on Syed and without the ability to rewind time, it's a difficult job to do. Even if I could travel back in time to the moments or hours that preceded the crime, there are no medical tests that can confirm the presence or absence of a 'mental illness' or 'personality disorder'. If only it were as easy as looking at an X-ray or taking a blood or urine sample, the analysis of which would show you exactly what sort of 'thing' you were dealing with. But there are no physical signposts to turmoil in the human psyche.

I had come prepared with an interview schedule and a host of mental health-related questionnaires and personality ratings scales to help me weigh up, in my professional judgement, whether or not Michael gave a credible description of having had thoughts, feelings and perceptions unusual enough to 'substantially impair' his criminal responsibility. Given that these phenomena are fleeting, intangible and open to interpretation, it's a little like trying to capture and then examine snowflakes in the palms of your hands. And all while trying to draw the line between normality and abnormality, if indeed such a line can be drawn.

Determining who is and who is not 'normal' is a contentious business. A weighty tome called the *Diagnostic and Statistical Manual of Mental Disorders* (or *DSM*, though I prefer to call it the *Big Book of Human Suffering*) is purportedly the ultimate guide to glitches of the mind and is used around the world by mental-health professionals, researchers, psychiatric drug regulation industries, health-insurance companies, pharmaceutical companies and so on. It has been published and updated by the American Psychiatric Association since 1952 and is now in its fifth edition. Revisions are agreed on by a clique of psychiatrists who decide by committee which mental 'disorders' should be included (it wasn't until 1973 that they dropped homosexuality). They also dictate which handy 'new' diagnoses to incorporate (growing from 128 categories in the first edition to a current whopping 541. Like Barnum's circus, the *DSM* has something for everybody).

As you may have guessed, I'm not a fan of the *Big Book of Human Suffering,* although it makes a great office doorstop. For starters, the vast majority of these (overwhelmingly white, male) committee members have declared financial ties to the pharmaceutical industry. It doesn't take a bloodhound to sniff out the unpalatable whiff of a potential conflict of interest here. Moreover, you would expect a diagnostic manual that is so influential to have developed out of a massive research effort; it actually has very little science to back it up. And I'm far from the only sceptic. The *DSM* has generated a raft of criticism over the years, perhaps none more damning than from one of its own creators.

In 2010, Professor Allen Frances, who was stepping down after being lead editor of the fourth edition, told a startled journalist, 'There is no definition of a mental disorder. It's bullshit. I mean, you just can't define it.' He went on, 'These concepts are virtually impossible to define precisely with bright lines at the boundaries.'

In 2019, an analysis of some of the diagnostic categories published in *Psychiatry Research* concluded that they were 'scientifically meaningless' (which is a technical term for 'bullshit'). They found so many hugely overlapping symptoms specified for different conditions that there are a possible 'one quintillion symptom combinations – more than stars in the Milky Way' that would meet criteria for the seven most commonly made diagnoses. What that means in practice is that two people can be given the same diagnostic label without having anything in common – or, like Michael, can see five different psychiatrists and end up with four different diagnoses.

If you are confused, then spare a thought for me, tasked with mapping these 'scientifically meaningless' and constantly evolving psychiatric constructs onto stagnant but equally mystifying legal definitions. Diagnostic labels tell us little about the individual concerned but they are the accepted and expected language of my work.

*

Michael slumped into the chair opposite me, acknowledging me with a curt nod and stretching his long legs out in front of him. He had put on a little weight since the photograph that earned him the 'baby-faced killer' moniker had been taken, possibly a side-effect of the olanzapine he'd been prescribed, one of the newer anti-psychotic medications. The extra few pounds accentuated the child-like quality of his face, which seemed somehow to be at odds with the rest of his body.

As I started to set out the reason for my visit, cautioning Michael that I would be taking detailed notes during our conversations that might be requested by the court, he let out a loud sigh. I didn't really blame him. After being assessed by a string of psychiatrists, he was probably bored to tears of repeating himself. But when a look of such sheer contempt flashed across his face, I found myself momentarily irritated. *When you've sat across the table from as many doctors as I have homicide defendants* then *you can get sniffy,* I thought to myself. *I'm not here for my own benefit.*

'Bradling.' He said the name through gritted teeth, as though it tasted salty. 'Bradling says I'm lying. I'm not a liar.'

'And I'm not Dr Bradling,' I replied. 'We don't work together and we form our opinions completely independently of each other. I'm here to get as much information as I can and listen to whatever you have to tell me. I have not arrived with any opinion.'

He nodded and the muscle in his jaw softened a little.

We started to work through my list of areas to explore, following a logical progression through Michael's life so far, including family structure and relationships, childhood experiences, school and employment history and so on. The idea is to work carefully up to the moments around and during the crime, which should then be deconstructed with the interviewee in fine detail.

One of the obvious problems with this type of assessment is that I am largely – although not entirely – reliant on what a person chooses to share with me. A defendant in a murder case has every incentive not to tell me the full story. The opinions and emotions they express in an interview are often carefully designed to suit the circumstances they are in or to shore up whatever forlorn hopes they may hold for the outcome of my report.

Michael told me he had no history of any type of abuse and that he'd never been involved in unlawful, reckless or cruel behaviour as a child. He told me he'd grown up in a stable, nurturing home, which perfectly echoed his mother's statement. He was well provided for and always enjoyed a good relationship with his stepfather, who had been a consistent figure in his life since he was a toddler. In short, there was nothing particularly revealing about Michael's early development and nor was there any available evidence to suggest his account was untrue.

Michael had left home to start basic training at Commando Training Centre Royal Marines in Devon at 16. 'Best time of my life,' he said, tapping his heart with his fist, 'getting that green beret.' Then he'd joined a Commando Unit as a rifleman.

'It didn't work out,' he said, and the muscle in his jaw started to set again.

'How come?'

'I just didn't like it,' he said, lips pursed. 'So I packed it in.'

He leaned back in his seat, folding his arms in a silent confirmation that this line of enquiry had hit a brick wall.

There was clearly more to this story. His mother had described how he was sullen and uncommunicative when he returned home, spending most of his time alone in his bedroom. He was bad-tempered at times, too, though there's nothing unusual in that from a teenage boy, particularly one with nothing to do.

I wanted to question Michael further about his departure from the Marines but I didn't have the rapport with him that the subject needed, or the time. My brief was very clear: I had to focus on Michael's circumstances at the time of the offences.

'What was your life like after you came out of the military?'

He said he enrolled at college and that was when 'it' started. He pulled up his T-shirt, pointing to two jagged silver-white scars on his abdomen.

'Jihadists.'

'Jihadists?'

'Yes, they put something in my blood, a sort of tracker. I could feel it moving through my body, making me sick in my stomach.'

Delusions are fantastical and strongly held beliefs. Although on the surface they may appear too surreal to understand, over the years I've come to make more sense of them by viewing them as growing out of a person's most deeply held needs or fears. Delusions are not necessarily unpleasant for the person experiencing them. Those involving themes of grandiosity and religion – becoming convinced that you are the Queen of Sheba, chosen by God or have special powers – can compensate nicely for a long-held sense of unimportance. At the other end of the spectrum, thoughts of persecution – believing you are under surveillance or threat of attack – can be downright horrific. For example, I once had to coax a petrified woman out of her attic. She thought her family had been replaced by aliens who were trying to take control of her mind and, in an effort to stop them, she was threatening to take a drill to her temple as she hid in the rafters.

The scars on Michael's stomach were the result of him cutting himself with a razor blade, he told me. 'I thought I could bleed it out of me but I couldn't. Then they started talking to me. Sometimes they took the mick out of me, called me a "soft bastard". They wanted me to join their holy war.'

'That sounds frightening, how did you deal with that?'

'I told them to fuck off! But they kept on at me, so I bargained with them, made a deal. They told me to kill someone. If I made a sacrifice to their holy war, they'd be satisfied and leave me alone.'

'That's a huge decision to take. Did you struggle with it?'

Michael leaned towards me and held his palms open. 'No. I didn't need to. It was easy. I knew when I joined the

Marines that I'd have to kill someone at some point, so what's the big deal?'

I was interested to see how Michael would behave when he recounted the moments leading up to the attacks and the step-by-step details of how he killed Finbar and attempted to murder Syed. Quite often, you almost have to drag a person through this stage of the interview. I've watched clients develop an anxiety rash before my eyes, shake uncontrollably, become selectively deaf, mute or both and even fall asleep. All of those reactions were a result of the person finding it unbearable to describe the truth of what they did. But that couldn't be said for Michael. In the same dry way he gave his statements to the police, he took me through every last detail of how he had killed Finbar.

When he described the way he slit his throat three times, so deep that the knife hit the man's spine, he could have been telling me how he'd chopped a tough and slippery parsnip for the Sunday roast.

Was there a hint of a self-satisfied smile on his face? I asked myself.

Michael told me he'd ruled out looking for a victim in the park closest to his home so as to avoid being recognized by potential witnesses. The park he settled on had more places to hide if a quick getaway was needed. When he almost immediately came across Finbar lying on the grass, he'd congratulated himself on his choice.

I wanted to know why he'd made an initial, superficial stab at Finbar's chest. It had struck me as an experimental 'tease' cut, which was at odds with the determined assault on the man's neck.

'Well, I'd never killed anybody before. I just wanted to see what his reaction was.'

'And?'

'He looked at me and screamed. It was…interesting,' he shrugged.

'Did it give you any second thoughts about what you were doing?'

'No. The voices were saying, "Go on, go on, do it, do it." So I got on with it.'

He described how he heard high-pitched, hysterical laughter in his head as he cut into Finbar's throat.

The victim made a gurgling noise, which filled Michael with an overwhelming urge to 'do something to stop him speaking evil about me'. It was then that he stuffed part of his coat in his mouth, pushing it as far down his gullet as he could.

'Speak evil to who?'

'I don't know, I can't explain it. To God maybe…it was just a strange feeling.'

I wondered if this was an indication of shame or remorse. He'd just killed a man, after all. But Michael claimed he felt nothing of the sort.

'Everyone wants to know if I feel sorry. I've tried to feel something but I can't. It was him or me, so I chose me. The guy was just collateral damage. The only thing I've lost sleep over is that I cocked up with the second one.'

Michael told me how, in the days leading up to his attack on Syed, the voices had 'wanted another one'. He'd found a housing estate with a wooded area at the perimeter, no visible CCTV and well away from where he'd killed Finbar. The ideal spot, he thought.

He intended to slit Syed's throat and 'cut his tongue out' but he said he'd made the mistake of taking a 'cheap knife'. 'Packing the wrong equipment is a schoolboy error,' he said.

I asked him why he chose Syed.

'I'm no racist!' he said, suddenly becoming very animated and pointing emphatically with his finger. 'He was just in the wrong place at the wrong time...' A smirk spread across his face as he considered his last statement. 'Wrong place and time for him, not me.'

'Is there anybody that you wouldn't have tried to kill if they had been out alone at that time?'

'What, you mean like women and kids?'

I nodded and he thought for a brief second. 'Probably not,' he shrugged.

I spent a total of six hours with Michael over two visits. There were moments when some of the detail, and the blunt way he delivered it, made the hairs on the back of my neck prickle. Even so, I felt that the more time we spent together the better we communicated; the contempt and distrust he had shown me at the start of our meeting began to thaw a little and, as we picked through the details of his life, Michael gradually became more open with me. Towards the end of the second interview, he told me he felt positive the medication he was now prescribed by his psychiatrist was 'in his bloodstream, blocking the tracker from working'. He also explained that the voices had less of a hold over him now and they had almost disappeared.

'The thing I don't understand,' he said, 'is that in a way, I miss them.' Glancing around the room, he added, 'They'd be a bit of company in this shithole, at least.'

All of a sudden, he looked like a lost teenage boy.

Without realizing it, Michael had given me a valuable piece of information, hitting on the fact that hearing voices is not always the torture or curse people assume it is. For some, it's a comfort and for many others, it's a conflicting mixture of both. If he were lying, it would be unlikely he would make this up, as it's a reaction to hearing voices few malingerers know about.

I'd had a couple of weeks to ponder my interviews with Michael, score up all my standardized personality and mental health-related ratings scales, and write up my report. It ran to 47 pages.

I was now sitting around an oversized oak table with the CPS lawyer, two junior solicitors and two of the investigating police officers. Each had a copy of my report in front of them, and a very serious expression on their face. The CPS lawyer – a well-groomed 40-something woman with a glossy crown of black hair – was a naturally warm and cheerful person. The first time we met she had reminded me of a contented cat, but today her eyes were boring like laser beams into the document. Her two junior solicitors – both young and female – wore suits as sombre as their faces and the two middle-aged police officers – one male, one female – looked like they were about to read somebody their rights. In unison, they began turning to the all-important 'opinion' section at the back. They would go through the whole report with a fine-tooth comb later, I hoped.

'So, what did you make of him, Kerry?' the CPS lawyer asked. 'Is he mad or bad?'

I didn't blame her for cutting to the chase. It was the question on everybody's lips and the reason I'd been brought in. Was the defendant lying about hearing voices or not? As the CPS lawyer had told me right at the start: 'We need this argument resolved and we know you don't sit on the fence, Kerry.'

'I think he's a bit of both…'

Every person around the table looked up from their reading and cocked their head to one side, like a synchronized swimming team. For a very brief moment, I felt like I *was* sitting on a fence, a pretty spiky and uncomfortable one at that. I didn't let their bemused expressions put me off my stride.

'Although rather than mad and bad,' I added firmly, 'I prefer to describe him as disturbed and disturbing.'

'That's inconvenient,' one of the police officers said under his breath. He tugged at his grey beard, dislodging a crumb that tumbled onto the front of his white shirt. He'd had burned toast for breakfast, by the looks of it, and his day was not getting any better.

'I can't find any evidence to suggest the defendant is lying about hearing voices,' I continued. 'What evidence there is supports Michael's story that he was influenced by command hallucinations to kill, in combination with some pretty disturbing persecutory delusions. He believed he was being tracked and targeted by jihadists. Although he was fully aware that what he was doing was illegal, by his logic he was defending himself against the threat. In legal terms, most people would consider this as an "abnormal" state of mind and that the experience was intense and distressing enough to impair both his reasoning and his willpower.'

The CPS lawyer trained her sharp eyes on mine, as if daring me to blink first.

'So you are saying he has a case for diminished responsibility?'

'Yes. In the end, that is what I am saying.'

The collective disappointment in the room was palpable. The bearded police officer was the first to challenge me.

'If he was mentally ill at the time, why were the assaults so calculated? Surely every bit of his behaviour would have been haywire and confused?'

This man has obviously never watched A Beautiful Mind, I thought.

'I grant you that a person's thinking can become highly disorganized when they are in an extreme state, but everyone is different. Michael, like a lot of people who live with psychosis, is not only intelligent and able to achieve much, he is capable of coherent planning.'

'But he was so precise in the way he cut Finbar Jackson's throat!' The police officer prodded the desk with his index finger, though I'm sure he wanted to point it straight at me. 'If he was psychotic, as you say, surely his aim would have been off?'

I kept my professional face on. The officer was only saying what a lot of people fortunate enough not to know much about mental-health problems might imagine.

'I can honestly say that I've never heard of hearing voices affecting anyone's hand–eye coordination,' I said politely.

'But you said he was *both* mad and bad,' the officer scowled. 'So you basically agree with Dr Bradling, that he is a psychopath?' He turned to his colleague, a slight, earnest-looking woman. 'We found him chilling when we interviewed him, didn't we?' She widened her small blue eyes and nodded keenly in agreement.

'It's true that Michael has worryingly callous, unemotional personality traits,' I said, 'but he hasn't demonstrated the turbulent relationships, disruptive and irresponsible behaviours needed to earn a confident diagnosis.'

I explained that the gold-standard assessment of psychopathy in a court of law is the Hare Psychopathy Checklist. There is a Youth Version, believe it or not, which is a 20-item rating scale of where 12- to 18-year-olds lie on the psychological and behavioural features of psychopathy. I'd had to put aside all my personal thoughts about a measure that can brand children as 'psychopaths' to carry out this assessment on Michael.

When I was writing up my report, I'd thought about

his military career, short though it was. Dr Kevin Dutton, research fellow at Oxford University and co-author of *The Good Psychopath's Guide to Success,* argues that the flagship features of a 'psychopathic personality' are necessary to get ahead in a number of careers. In the Marines, Michael's focus, his ability to switch aggression on at will and his skill at making quick, ruthless decisions would have all been feathers in his cap. The same characteristics were viewed very differently when he chose to kill one man and left another fighting for his life. It's only in that context that Michael's personality had come to be seen as 'disordered'.

'The line between a good psychopath and a bad psychopath can be vanishingly thin,' Dr Dutton says. According to his research, some of the highest levels of psychopathic traits can be found in journalists, CEOs, surgeons, lawyers and police officers. Given the company I was in, I decided not to share that little nugget.

I told the meeting there was one thing Dr Bradling and I could agree on: Michael's more unpleasant personality characteristics did not 'substantially impair' his responsibility for the crimes. But for me, I explained, it was the *interaction* between his personality and his troubled mental state that was significant. When a willingness to kill becomes coupled with a reason to kill – no matter how bizarre or deluded that reason may be – the results are catastrophic.

At this point, one of the junior solicitors summed things up neatly. 'Are you saying a person can be a bit of a psychopath and psychotic at the same time?'

'They can indeed,' I replied. 'That is exactly what I'm saying. Although it is the presence of voices and delusional beliefs that are legally relevant in this case.'

Now it was the CPS lawyer's turn to say, 'That's inconvenient,' but she didn't mutter it under her breath like the officer had. She said it out loud, prompting a bob of heads from the synchronized swimming team.

A few days later I received a phone call from the CPS lawyer. After due consideration, the Crown would not be accepting Michael's diminished responsibility plea to the murder and attempted murder charges. The matter would be left for a jury to decide. The lawyer didn't owe me an explanation but she launched into one nonetheless, sounding almost apologetic. There had been a huge amount of interest in Michael's case, from both the public and the media, she said. Speculation that the attack on Syed was racially motivated had provoked terror and outrage in the community, and the police investigation had been large and expensive. I understood what she was really saying. The case was a political hot potato.

A person's right to be tried by a jury of their peers is a central principle of UK law. For that reason, I wasn't disappointed by the decision, though I admit I did wonder if Michael would be judged on the weight of the evidence alone, given the hype and heightened emotions his case had stirred up.

It put me in mind of the infamous case of Peter Sutcliffe. He had been diagnosed with 'paranoid schizophrenia' by four psychiatrists prior to his trial for killing 13 women (and attempting to kill seven others). The CPS intended to accept his plea of diminished responsibility, but the trial judge intervened, unusually, insisting that he be tried before a jury. They found Sutcliffe guilty of murder on all counts and he was eventually handed a whole-life sentence. However, when his mental state deteriorated, he was transferred out of prison to Broadmoor, a move that caused sections of the media to rage about his 'cushy' conditions. Secure hospitals, with their individual bedrooms and focus on therapy, are typically seen as 'justice lite' by those who have never set foot in one. Broadmoor is far from being the Savoy Hotel but some accused Sutcliffe of feigning mental distress to con his way inside and campaigns were mounted for him to be shipped back to prison and 'properly punished'.

It seemed to me that the CPS was working very hard in Michael's case to avoid a similar public backlash. They had to get it right, or at least to be seen to be doing so.

Dr Bradling would appear for the prosecution and slug it out with the four defence psychiatrists. My report would not see the light of day. Though I'd clearly set out my belief in Michael's 'abnormality of mind', not even the defence team was going to call me to give evidence. The fact that I'd also included a hard-to-swallow description of parts of Michael's personality would only confuse the jury. Courtroom battles work best with cut-and-dried arguments, and black-and-white snapshots of people are valued over 'inconvenient' full-colour portraits.

*

After a two-week trial, it took the jury just over a day to reach its verdict. Just like the prosecution team, the members of the jury had preferred the opinion of Dr Bradling. Michael was simply a psychopath, they decided. He was found guilty of murder and attempted murder.

On the day of Michael's sentencing, I was at a solicitor's office adjacent to the Crown Court he had been tried in. It was pouring down with rain as I ran up the wide stone steps, trying not to splatter too much dirty water up the back of my trouser legs. The judge was in the middle of his summing up when I crammed myself into a wooden bench at the side of the packed courtroom.

'The jury had to consider all of the evidence, not just the expert evidence. In particular, the jury had to assess the truthfulness of your claim to have been acting under the compulsion of voices you were hearing. The jury rejected your defence of diminished responsibility.'

I was looking at Michael, who was staring straight ahead. He began picking his fingers as the judge continued his summing up, describing how the case against him had been made worse by the brutal nature of the stabbings and the public anxiety the murder and attempted murder had caused.

'As Dr Bradling put it, your judgement may be considered illegal, immoral and abhorrent but it was based on nothing more than a desire to kill and was entirely rational. Two of the psychiatrists called by the defence acknowledged on the stand that if they were wrong about psychosis, the only other explanation for such atrocious acts is that you must be a psychopath. You are a deceiver and a manipulator and you have *lied* about hearing voices.'

The damning words crashed off the wood-panelled walls. I didn't take my eyes off Michael for a second. He shook his head almost imperceptibly as the judge delivered the last line, emphasizing the word 'lied' with considerable aplomb.

The judge ordered Michael to his feet for sentencing. He obliged, albeit belligerently, dragging himself off his seat.

'For the offences of murder and attempted murder you will be detained at Her Majesty's Pleasure. That is the same as a sentence of life imprisonment. You will serve a minimum term of 21 years, less the 412 days you have spent on remand. Thereafter, it will be for the parole board to decide when, if ever, you should be released.'

'I don't give a flying fuck.'

Michael dropped the words from his half-closed mouth. They were almost lost in the ripple of applause that broke out in the public gallery in response to his life sentence but there was no mistaking what he'd said.

Syed Akbar was on the front row of the public gallery, flanked by his wife and daughter. He looked shell-shocked rather than jubilant. He had gone through the ordeal of this trial, no doubt hoping to find answers. I wondered if it had been cathartic in any way and found myself doubting it. All the man had learned was that he had been attacked by a stranger for no reason, other than that the stranger was a murderous psychopath. How do you ever make sense of that? It seemed a very inadequate explanation to me.

*

Some years later, I was in the healthcare unit of a maximum-security prison, having visited an inmate for an assessment. A female prison officer was escorting me out through a wing flanked with cells and side dorms lined with hospital beds. I was looking forward to getting out of there and reaching the peace and quiet of my car. Healthcare units, known as 'Fraggle Rock' in prison slang, can be chaotic, filled with all the sounds and smells of the jungle. This one was no exception. Frantic cries of 'Nurse! Nurse!' and 'Where's me fuckin' drugs!' rang through the air while the smell of sterilizing fluid mixed with stale sweat and bad guts was clinging to my nostrils.

Two inmates were singing the England football song 'Vindaloo' at the top of their lungs, taking it in turns to shout out the rhyming lines about cheddar cheese, please, Waterloo and a bucket of vindaloo. At the chorus, they went full throttle, belting out the 'nah nah nahs' through the barred gates of their adjacent cells. This medley had been going on for half the morning and was getting on my last nerve. Still, for once I hadn't had any lewd remarks slung at me, a rarity in an environment like this. *Be thankful for small mercies*, I thought, preparing to be handed back my handbag and car keys and breathe some fresh air.

To reach the exit, the prison officer had to take me past a row of safe cells, the sort fitted with concealed fixtures and seamless, round-edged furniture that are used for prisoners at high risk of self-harm or suicide. That's when I heard something that cut through the cocktail of sounds, giving me a sharp mental jolt.

'I don't give a flying fuck!'

I took a few more steps, stopped at the next safe cell and looked inside. He was well into his twenties by now, but I recognized him immediately.

'Hello, Michael,' I said. 'Do you remember me?'

He seemed to look straight through me. His face was slimmer than before, his jaw had squared off and he had a wispy half-attempt at a beard. His skin had a strange hue, like a faded Post-it note.

'I'm Kerry Daynes, a psychologist. I came to see you in hospital, before your trial.'

He shook his head and turned away.

'Don't bother about him, love,' the prison officer said. 'He's always like that. He's always stopping and starting his meds.'

Michael was in a safe cell because he had been cutting himself.

'He thinks all the terrorists in the place are trying to recruit him,' the prison officer explained, shaking her head and giving a derisory little snort. 'He's been digging into his stomach with the end of a sharpened toothbrush.'

Another day and another fuck-up, I thought. An image of the expensively attired and unshakably confident Dr Bradling flashed into my mind. How would he react if he were standing beside me, looking at this so-called liar, still desperate to bleed the tracker out of his body?

Does it really matter, you might think, *as long as a killer is safely behind bars?* But I have to question if Michael was any less dangerous in the long term, given that he had become just one of the thousands of prison inmates who struggle with severe mental-health problems in an institution ill-equipped to provide the level of support he needed.

In *They Say You're Crazy,* clinical psychologist Paula Caplan writes that naming something is an act of power. Particularly, she says, when it comes to classifying and labelling an aspect of a person, or their entire personality, as 'disordered'. In a court of law, the ramifications of getting it wrong are enormous and that power should weigh heavily on any professional expert.

I walked in silence with the prison officer as she guided me through several metal gates back to the prison reception. Standing in the air lock, the last obstacle separating me from the outside world, I once again mulled over Michael's brief stint in the Marines. What on earth had caused him to walk away from the career that he'd trained so hard for? I'd never know. It seemed to me that a critical part of his journey towards becoming a killer lay buried. Had it been found, would the missing piece of the jigsaw have persuaded Dr Bradling or the jury to see Michael as more than a straight-up, deviant murderer?

Maybe. Then again, maybe not.

The reality is that life and people are complicated. And the judgements made in legal settings are more subjective, unscientific and driven by media stories, popular perceptions and misconceptions than we might care to admit. The bright line that we draw between 'madness' and 'badness' can be genuinely blinding, and yet it doesn't really exist.

CHAPTER TWO

DO NO HARM

My new client looked like a piece of paper that had been scrunched into a ball and then smoothed out again.

'It's Clifford, not Cliff,' he said resolutely, by way of introducing himself.

'Pleased to meet you,' I smiled. 'I'm Kerry.'

Clifford not Cliff had an unruly beard, a mop of morning hair and was wearing a creased, oversized raincoat, unironed shirt and a pair of trousers that seemed at least four sizes too big for him. In one hand he carried a bulging brown leather satchel, in the other a Tesco carrier bag with a packet of crumpets poking out of the top.

The venue for our meeting was his solicitor's office, a single-storey building that stood alone in the middle of a Bolton shopping precinct. It was the sort of place that looked like it might have been a Timpson's shoe-repair shop in a former life and to reach the single office you had to squeeze through a reception area the size of a broom cupboard. Floor-to-ceiling shelving crammed with box files and a mismatched collection of filing cabinets occupied most of the room, and unfiled paperwork was stacked in neat towers on patches of the carpet-tiled floor. *You couldn't swing a cat in here*, I thought, but at least I was faring better than the receptionist, who must have felt like a battery hen.

There was a desk in front of the far wall, although, 'far' was something of a misnomer. Having arrived first, I'd taken the chair to the side of the desk and left the padded leather armchair at the back – the obvious 'power seat' – for Clifford. It's something I often try to do with clients, so they feel a little less like they are at an extended GP appointment or back in the head teacher's office.

Clifford had quite an imposing physical presence, filling what little space was left in the room. 'I'm sorry I haven't had time to trim my beard this morning,' he apologized, stroking his chin before manoeuvring into his chair.

I'd heard a faint jangle of metal as soon as he had come through the door. Now I saw that there were chains attached to his belt, from which dangled his wallet, keys and a pocket diary. Interesting sartorial choices, I thought.

'I was in London until late last night,' he went on. 'Lobbying Parliament on a housing matter.' He puffed out his broad chest as he imparted this piece of information.

This was the first of two meetings we had scheduled, due to the fact Clifford was a fan of the 'five-finger discount'. Or, to put it another way, he was a repeat shoplifter.

It was 2003 and I was still in my twenties (just), working three days a week at a medium-secure hospital and two days a week in my newly established private practice, which was busy from the word go. I'd recently landed my first contract to supply psychology services at the forensic step-down project, Laurel House, I was increasingly being asked to consult in police investigations and there were plenty of others who wanted my advice. The majority of my referrals were from solicitors asking for assessments of their clients for use at various stages of criminal-court proceedings. It was three years before I would work on Michael's contentious case but right from the start, my in-tray was brimming with homicide, sexual abuse and assault cases. In between the intense and thorny work that came in, I was happy to take on comparatively mundane jobs like this one. An assessment of a petty offender might not seem exciting but 'excitement' in the world of forensic psychology has a habit of turning you into a gibbering mess by the end of the day. This was my bread-and-butter work and I was grateful for it.

The letter of instruction from Clifford's solicitor told me that a report was potentially needed for two looming court cases. The first was an appeal against a conviction at Bolton Magistrates' Court for stealing six folding umbrellas and a tube of hand cream from a branch of Boots, for which Clifford had been handed a 12-month Community Rehabilitation Order and ordered to pay £200 costs. Secondly, Clifford stood accused of stealing six travel alarm clocks from British Home Stores in Blackpool. What anyone would want with six folding umbrellas and six travel alarm clocks was a mystery in itself, I thought, even without a question mark over Clifford's psychological state.

'My client intends to vigorously contest both matters,' the solicitor wrote. 'He maintains that he has memory problems and simply forgot to pay for the said goods. I therefore require you to confine your report strictly to an assessment of my client's memory capacity.'

When I'd telephoned to request a copy of Clifford's medical records, my usual procedure even for such a bog-standard assessment as this, the solicitor had informed me, with an ominously weary sigh, that he doubted very much that his client would give permission, but he would brace himself to ask.

I explained to Clifford that the purpose of today's appointment was for me to collect as much information as I could to get an overview of how well, or otherwise, his memory had been performing for him these past 43 years. When we met again in two weeks' time, I would assess his current memory skills more formally by taking him through a standardized series of tests.

'Right you are, Katie,' he said in his mild Mancunian accent. Clifford had started to make notes in his pocket book and I spotted that he'd written my name down as Katie.

'It's Kerry,' I corrected. 'K-E-R-R-Y.'

'Ah, right. Thank you for pointing that out. Before we start, I want to show you some of my paperwork.'

He opened his satchel and started rifling through reams of paper, pulling out photocopies of job applications, letters to the *Bolton Evening News* and the Crown Prosecution Service and copies of correspondence addressed to the 'criminal justice system' until they were scattered all over the desk, adding to the already suffocating feeling of the room.

'Here we go,' he said, handing me a couple of sheets. 'Proof that I am being persecuted by the state, Katie.'

It was a copy of a witness statement from the Loss Prevention Officer (aka the store detective) at British Home Stores in Blackpool.

'I observed the man placing a travel alarm clock into each pocket of his raincoat and two into each of his trouser pockets. He had attracted my attention as his trousers were unusually baggy and were tucked into his boots and tied around the ankles with laces.'

I felt the side of my lips start to quiver as I suppressed a smile. As he was 'clocked' by the store detective, Clifford must have been ticking louder than the crocodile in *Peter Pan*.

The store detective went on to say that Clifford left the store without paying, was approached outside, brought back in and searched. Two clocks were found in his raincoat pockets and the other four around his ankles, captured inside the legs of his tied-up trouser bottoms. His trouser pockets were found to be 'adapted', the bottom of both having been deliberately cut out. *No wonder his wallet and keys were on chains*, I thought.

The statement went on to explain that Clifford had been immediately issued with a town exclusion order, barring him from entering the high street, which he'd loudly refused to sign. Whereupon the police were called and charges pressed.

I hadn't asked but Clifford volunteered the fact he'd been in Blackpool 'celebrating'.

'I won a compensation case,' he said proudly. 'I was awarded £150 after being bitten by a basset hound outside Tesco Express. I was having a good day until Officer Dibble and his mates grabbed me.'

Ever a sucker for an eccentric, I was warming to Clifford, even if he was a one-man crime wave.

Another witness statement told me he had been stopped in Boots after their store manager saw him stuffing the six umbrellas in his 'pockets'. It was a similar story, with three found bunched around each ankle.

Oh Clifford, I thought to myself, *you have all the subtlety and guile of three chipmunks in a trenchcoat!*

'I have been used and abused by a corrupt so-called justice system,' he announced, blowing out a wayward hair that had strayed from his beard into his mouth. 'And when your report declares me an innocent man I will be demanding they get on their knees and apologize.'

'Just hold on a moment,' I interrupted.

It was time to manage Clifford's expectations before he got too carried away. What is known in law as 'the ultimate question' – whether a defendant is guilty or innocent – is not for me to decide. The role of a psychologist is simply to provide evidence, for the court not the client, and to avoid sailing too close to offering an opinion that might steal a judge or jury's thunder. So if Clifford was under the impression that I was there as his hired gun, he was about to learn otherwise.

'My report won't make any comment about your guilt or innocence. That is not my job.' Clifford's shoulders started to sag. 'I'm just here to use my expertise to collect the most accurate information possible. If your solicitor thinks that it will be helpful, it will be given to the court but it is up to them what they make of it alongside the rest of the evidence, OK?'

And good luck with that, I mused, wondering how on earth someone with holes cut in his pockets and string wrapped around the bottom of his trouser legs could possibly claim that they merely forgot to pay. Mind you, as my Irish relatives always say, God loves a trier.

'The courts are full of nincompoops!' Clifford protested.

'Well, let's try our best to give them a clear and complete assessment that even a nincompoop can understand, then, shall we?' He nodded begrudgingly. 'Good, I've got lots of questions that I need to ask you, so let's crack on with it.'

We began working our way through my list of screening questions – where did you go to school? Have you ever had a head injury or been knocked unconscious? What jobs have you had? Have you ever taken illegal drugs? Basic things that most of us, being experts on our own lives, would breeze through. Clifford was able to tell me that he was unemployed at the moment and living in a flat where he was secretary of the Tenants' Association. He said he drank precisely four pints of beer on Thursday nights in the Nag's Head and visited his elderly mother every fortnight, but anything about his past, even the simplest historical facts, seemed to tax him.

'Now, let me think,' he said every time I tried to get him to turn the clock back to his earlier life. 'I can't remember that far back, so I'm not sure I can answer that question.' He seemed genuinely frustrated and disappointed in himself, not to be any more help.

'What about your mental health?' I asked. 'Have you ever found yourself struggling with that?' This was a reasonable question and hopefully one he might manage to answer.

Clifford thought long and hard. 'I wouldn't have thought so,' he said noncommittally, before changing the subject.

'I want you to have a look at some more of these,' he said, plucking a couple of photocopied sheets of paper off the desk. Now he was the one steering the conversation, Clifford's shoulders lifted and he seemed much more confident.

I did as he instructed. I think I'd worn him out for the time being and, besides, the most unlikely segues in a conversation have a habit of telling you more than an entire catalogue of prompts and probes often can.

'Read these first, Katie,' he said, nodding his head in encouragement.

If Clifford had trouble remembering the most basic information about himself, what hope did he have of remembering my name? I'd just have to resign myself to being Katie, I realized. Still, I've answered to a lot worse.

Dear Criminal 'Justice' System,
Again I request that you drop this tiny matter in the public interest. You should be pursuing the real criminals with more vigour. I am a graduate of Manchester University and a well-respected, civic-minded person and pursuing me will be perceived as a vindictive, cruel, unjust and discriminatory act by the state.

I was not able to attend your wonderful court due to a mix up with dates and you imprisoned me for three days on remand and ruined my bank holiday weekend.

I had to share a very uncomfortable cell with a potentially dangerous person who had questionable personal hygiene.

I have been punished enough. I shall be taking this case of oppression by the state to my member of Parliament. Please drop this case now and apologize for harassing a respectable man.

Who elected the Crown, the monarchy and the nits who run the country and the backward, almost fascist criminal courts? Certainly not me, or anyone in Bronte Court Tenants Association.

This is costing me a lot of time and getting in the way of me pursuing employment opportunities.

Yours sincerely,

Clifford M Booth

'I can see that this is a difficult situation for you,' I said diplomatically, 'and I see that you went to Manchester University, tell me about your degree.'

Clifford said he had a first-class degree in sociology. However, he couldn't shed a single beam of light on any of his student days, looking blank and confused when he failed to answer my queries about where he'd lived and the friends he'd made. There was no amusing story to share about the state of his student digs or that time he'd lived on baked beans and cheap lager for six months. It was just like earlier, when he'd told me the name of the secondary school he'd attended in Bolton but couldn't describe his time there, his favourite subjects or give any hint as to what he was like as a teenager.

'It was a long time ago' he said. 'Does anybody remember their first day at university?'

'Yes, they mostly do,' I replied. 'It's unusual not to remember these things, Clifford.'

We all have autobiographical memory. In *The Memory Illusion,* Dr Julia Shaw calls it 'our personal memory scrapbook; our mind's diary; our internal Facebook timeline'.

It is this particular memory store that helps us understand our life trajectories and defines who we are. Personally, I think of it as an intricate piece of fabric: the threads of our own recollections interwoven with memories our parents have shared with us, photographs we've seen and events we've been a part of and elaborated on in the re-telling. All of these threads – some as thin as cobwebs, others as strong as fishermen's rope – are knitted into the tapestry of our past, creating an internal life story we keep on weaving.

For most people, out of a lifetime of collected memories, those created between the ages of 10 and 30 remain the strongest threads. But in Clifford's case, his autobiographical memory was more like a moth-eaten string vest than an elaborate embroidery. It meant I was having a hard time knowing quite what to believe. Did his sociology degree and the Bronte Court Tenants Association even exist, or were they nothing more than figments of this peculiar man's imagination?

'Tell me about the jobs that you've been applying for.'

Clifford gestured to the job-application forms among his paperwork and declared that he wanted to be a communist.

'Is being a communist an actual job?' I asked the question as politely as I could. 'I thought it was a political belief.'

He had no answer to that. 'I'd like to work for a trade union or as a researcher for an MP. I'm a socialist, you see, a politician. But the system isn't fair and they won't let me in. Sometimes I get interviews but I never get the job. It's discriminatory.'

Clifford told me he had been unemployed for as long as he could recall, around 20 years. When I asked what he did before that, perhaps after he left university, he couldn't tell me.

'The thing is, I could do much better than Tony Blair is doing. Or I could do Iain Duncan Smith's job.'

'The well-known socialist Iain Duncan Smith?' I quipped, given that the true-blue politician was the pro-hanging, pro-corporal punishment leader of the Conservative party at the time. Clifford nodded earnestly, clearly not getting the joke. That wiped the smile off my face. Despite my misgivings about his honesty, I liked Clifford and I certainly didn't want to ridicule him.

'It is unfair,' he said, shuffling his paperwork officiously. 'I'm always giving people advice about their tenancy agreement or employment rights but I never get any feedback or thanks for it. My skills are never recognized.'

For the rest of our meeting, it felt as though we went around in circles, Clifford banging his mutinous drum louder and louder to fill the silences that ensued whenever I tried to draw out the answers to my questions about his past. I could tell he felt irritated and perhaps a little embarrassed by the gaps in his history.

He conceded he was a little forgetful these days but he wrote down anything important in the notebook attached to his belt and managed 'just fine'. There were no problems with his concentration and attention span, of that he was certain, and it was only the false allegations of store detectives and the state that were standing between him and a glittering career in politics.

Understandably, pride may have been stopping him from acknowledging there was a problem but this in itself left me feeling baffled. Clifford was the antithesis of a wily criminal mastermind – unless I was falling for some sort of convoluted double bluff. He clearly hoped I would prove to the courts that he did indeed have a terrible memory, so why was he diverting my attention away from the black holes in his mind?

On the day of Clifford's second appointment, I arrived at the solicitor's office with a huge rucksack so full of equipment it made Clifford's packed satchel look slim. I was conducting the Wechsler Memory Scale, Third Edition, known as the WMS-III for short, though there is nothing short about it. It's a set of 11 subtests, each designed to assess 'clinically relevant aspects of memory functioning' and allow for comparison between the abilities of the person taking the test and others of the same age.

Just as I was having a last-minute study of the WMS-III technical manual, Clifford lurched into the room. He was sporting his Columbo-esque raincoat together with a splint on his right middle finger, an egg-shaped yellowing bruise on his forehead and a small graze on his nose. To cap it all, his hair was like Boris Johnson's in a force-nine gale.

'Hello, what happened to you?'

He told me had been thrown out of the pub on Thursday – literally, and at high speed – for 'talking too much politics'. And to add to the indignity of the situation, he'd only been part-way through pint number three.

'I will be seeking compensation and a full apology,' he assured me. I didn't doubt it.

'I've written to my probation officer. I was meant to have my first appointment with her this week but I'm sure you agree that there is no point in me going.' He handed me a copy of the letter from his satchel.

Dear Sandra,

Thank you for this appointment which I was looking forward to attending but will be unable to for the following reasons:

1.   I was badly assaulted at the Nags Head public house but the marvellous Greater Manchester police have failed to apprehend my assailants. I have a broken finger and a sore head and am unable to attend appointments et al for several weeks hence. Complaints against GMP for POOR QUALITY SERVICE are currently with Bolton police station and our local member of Parliament. Photos of injuries are enclosed.

2.   I was wrongfully found guilty of theft of £25.93

worth of goods from Boots. In a vindictive manner, the magistrates fined me £200 and gave me a Probation Order for 12 months. I should not have been in court that day, due to a heavy cold, but was forced there by the wonderfully fair and democratic 'justice' system.

3.   A full appeal has been lodged and complaints about my treatment will be made later following a no-doubt favourable report from Ms. Katie Daynes, my forensic psychologist.

4.   I have a good chance of securing employment as a trade union official and starting probation may put a black mark against my name. So therefore, please cancel the weekly probation meetings for now.

I have the pleasure of enclosing some socialist material, written by myself.

Yours sincerely,

Mr Clifford M Booth

Diploma in Social Policy, London, 1980

BA Honours, Sociology, Manchester University, 1983

PS Please write back to me as soon as possible.

I sympathized with Clifford about his injuries but I wasn't going to be drawn into aiding and abetting his skiving off probation appointments. Sandra, I could see, had quite enough to contend with already.

The WMS-III takes well over an hour to complete and is quite exhausting at the best of times, for both client and psychologist. So I told Clifford we'd better get started. There is an optional Information and Orientation subtest at the start that asks questions like 'What day of the month is this?' and 'Without looking at the clock, what time is it now?' It's fairly crude but is effective in identifying those who might have Alzheimer's or other memory-robbing diseases. At that stage in my career, dementia was the only thing I could think of that was capable of wiping out Clifford's autobiographical memories, although part of the cruelty of the illness is that fragments of a person's earliest memories remain the most intact, like a tapestry rescued from a fire, leaving them stranded and confused in that time period. This didn't fit with Clifford, who appeared to be very much in the here and now, with seemingly no past left to live in at all. Something wasn't adding up, so I was keen to hear his answers to these questions. Patterns of inconsistent performance on these simple questions can reveal someone who is faking; if Clifford was pulling the wool over my eyes, I felt certain I was about to outfox him.

But my confidence was misplaced. Clifford galloped through the questions entirely correctly, which only added to my puzzlement. Maybe he registered a look of surprise on my face. 'I'm not puddled, you know,' he said crossly, rolling his eyes.

'No,' I agreed. 'You are not.'

But as we ploughed on through the laborious assessment, Clifford's bravado started to wane. I read him a brief story about a woman called Anna Thompson from south London who was employed in a school canteen. 'She reported to the police that she'd been held up on a high street the night before and robbed of £56. She had four small children, the rent was due and they'd not eaten for two days. The police, touched by the woman's story, took up a collection for her.'

Immediately after reading it, I asked Clifford to repeat back to me as much as he could remember.

'I bet the police didn't take up a collection. I bet she had the bad service I always get.'

'No, Clifford. Please let's not get side-tracked. I just need you to tell me what you remember of the story.'

'I could help that woman! I could advise her! What sort of country do we live in?'

When I finally got him to focus, Clifford could relay scant details of the story.

Exactly 25 minutes later, I tested his delayed recall by asking him to remember everything he could about the story again, prompting him that 'it was about a woman who got robbed'. Beads of perspiration started to appear on his forehead and the end of his nose flushed pink. Clifford recalled only two of the 25 components of the story. 'I'm sorry,' he said, looking crestfallen.

At the end of the session, it was obvious that Clifford's ability to recall both verbal and visual information after a short time period was significantly below what would be predicted for a man of his age, and his immediate recall and working memory were barely hovering around average. Add to that his extremely threadbare autobiographical memory and Clifford was a conundrum – one beyond the scope of my expertise to solve. I felt it was necessary to provide his GP with a copy of the WMS-III test scores and let doctors investigate further. I explained this to Clifford.

'No, absolutely not,' he said, picking up his satchel and hugging it to him.

'Why not? I think that blood tests to rule out any illness, and maybe being seen by a neuropsychologist, could be really helpful in trying to get to the bottom of why you have some greater than expected problems with your memory.'

'No. I don't trust doctors.'

'How come?'

He thought for a moment. 'They are owned by the state. They are part of the corrupt Establishment.'

There was no changing his mind.

Our appointment was over. Before we said goodbye, I told him, 'With the best will in the world, I hope I don't see you under similar circumstances again, Clifford.' It's something I say to all my clients, though I don't always get my wish.

I wrote my report, limiting it, as instructed, to the issue of how Clifford's mind recalled information and detailing the nature of his very real memory deficits. I wished I could have provided a bigger picture but it was not for me to say if his memory problems were linked to his failure to pay for the goods found in his possession. Then again, I thought even a blindfolded mole would be able to see he had other motivations that coexisted with his memory problems.

Forgetful as he was, it was obvious Clifford was deliberately setting out to shoplift, and a desire for half a dozen folding umbrellas and travel alarm clocks was unlikely to be what propelled him. It seemed to me that his thievery was a directionless form of protest, a means of railing against the powers that be in a world that largely excluded him, rather than making space for his eccentricities. Clifford had a satchel full of causes, yet he was a rebel without any real cause, and not much of a clue.

I discovered later that Clifford won his appeal and was also cleared of the second shoplifting charge. It was a lesson in the power of a psychologist's report, one that didn't sit comfortably with me. Three headline words – 'significant memory deficits' – were ultimately all it took to get Clifford off the hook and a man who probably had the gall to go to court in his customized shoplifting trousers got off scot-free, or as free as he could be considering the load of other challenges he carried with him.

The courts are full of nincompoops, I thought to myself.

A couple of months after Clifford's legal victories, I handed in my notice at my hospital post and prepared to leave for a somewhat daunting future as a full-time, self-employed psychologist in private practice. I'd worked in secure hospitals, unlocking and locking doors behind me, for the past eight years but the post had made me fall out of love with this particular strand of my work.

The rot started to set in after one patient went temporarily

AWOL, making the news by attempting to go on the run in a tractor. The management team went into overdrive, implementing a damage-limitation strategy any politician would be proud of. They threw money at extra security measures and launched a glossy PR initiative designed to improve their reputation. Unfortunately, all of this was distracting from some real concerns about the quality of service on offer and behind the spruced-up facade neglect was rife. To say this led to disgruntlement among the staff is an understatement. It was incredibly irritating to see resources being pumped into fancy flowerbeds, new logos and mesh fencing while staff shortages, unnecessary bureaucracy and poor patient care were all being overlooked. We were disillusioned and angry. Every day brought fresh resentment.

The 'improved' security checks we had to go through just to get into and out of the grounds were exacted rigorously. One psychologist tried to pop in to check his emails but he had his dog in the car and was refused entry because the pooch didn't have valid identification. He was so hacked off he attempted to storm the painfully slow security barrier fitted at the gate, almost smashing straight through it at high speed. Meanwhile, stationery and loo rolls started disappearing from store cupboards and staff were signing themselves into the never-ending succession of meetings with names like 'Harry Azcrac' and 'Dixie Normous'. Puerile as it was, it was a way of raging against a system that the staff didn't respect or feel they had a say in.

On the subject of meetings, the head of psychology was refusing to attend our departmental meeting any more, due to our collective inability to ever make a decision. This torturous weekly event was chaired by my supervisor, a nurse with a love of dangly earrings who had retrained as a psychoanalytic therapist. We didn't see eye-to-eye at the best of times; suffice to say that we had vastly different approaches.

I believe that psychoanalysis has value, but when used sparingly alongside the more practical, relatable forms of therapeutic intervention that I instinctively lean to. Lying on a couch twice a week for five years, enduring long silences and someone else's interpretations of your relationship with your mother ('Oh, you don't agree? Perhaps we need to spend an additional year exploring your unconscious resistance to really connecting with this process, hmm?') just doesn't appeal to me. And I doubt very much that it appeals to anybody who is locked in a secure unit, praying that they might one day taste freedom while they still have their own teeth.

The supervisor and I had clashed over a new 'feminist initiative' that she'd introduced, which essentially consisted of rounding up the women patients every Friday and making them sing 'Sisters Are Doing It for Themselves'. Don't get me wrong, I love karaoke, but I had questioned how 'empowering' this actually was in an environment where the patients, the majority of whom had learning difficulties, were hardly allowed to make a single decision for themselves, even on a matter as harmless as a song choice.

My observation was not appreciated, though my

supervisor was not a stranger to making some unsolicited observations of her own.

'I notice you play with your hair,' she'd say. 'That has a deep psychological significance but I'm not going to tell you what it is.'

I know I twiddle my hair. It is a habit I formed when I was a child. I do it when I'm anxious because I find the action soothing, that's all.

She'd have a mysterious expression on her face, as I picked the bourbon and not the custard cream, as though she, and only she, had cracked the code to unlocking the secrets of the psyche.

'Sometimes a cigar is just a cigar,' I'd say, quoting Freud himself. Was it any wonder, under such tedious, navel-gazing leadership, that our department was in a state of near-paralysis?

Our already strained relationship had taken a turn for the worse one day when I drove from one side of the hospital site to the other, fresh from leading an anger-management group. I had two psychology assistants with me and was running late for my next session when a massive delivery truck (probably with another consignment of shiny brochures or perhaps a decorative water fountain) blocked my entrance to the car park.

'Stuff it,' I said to the two assistants. 'Only one thing for it.'

I drove up the grassy embankment to bypass the lorry. It wasn't my best-laid plan, not least because I'd only recently passed my test and was a terrible driver. The car ground to a halt on top of the bank and, even with my foot to the floor and the engine at full revs, it was going nowhere.

'Can you two push from the back?' I asked my colleagues.

Sarah and Rebecca jumped out and started pushing with all their might. The car wasn't budging and that's when I suddenly realized why. In my haste, I'd left the handbrake on. I immediately released it, at which point my mint-green Mini Cooper shot across the embankment like a runaway train and the two assistants landed face-down in the tyre-mangled grass.

We all thought it was hilarious and got on with our day, but the following week my supervisor called me into her office. My faux-pas had been captured on one of the swanky new CCTV cameras and shown to my self-satisfied supervisor.

'We have it all on camera and I've asked Sarah and Rebecca to write official statements,' she said. 'Is this something you would like to deny?'

'No! Of course not. I hold my hands up!'

She studied me frostily. 'It was a destructive act. Damage has been caused to the grass. Were you angry?'

'No!'

'You were coming from the anger-management group. Do you think you were acting out some unconscious feelings from the group?'

I couldn't believe she was making such a mountain out of a molehill, or even a small grassy embankment. I told her again that no, it was nothing of the sort. It was a momentary error of judgement, fuelled by my desire to arrive at my next group on time. No more, no less.

She and the chief executive had held (another) meeting and decided that I should pay £175 to replace the damaged grass.

Fair enough, I thought, although it seemed expensive. 'What kind of grass is this?' I asked. 'Are you going to plant it or smoke it?'

She looked at me with naked disdain and I smirked back insolently. It was official: we loathed each other.

When my moment came to finally wave goodbye to the hospital I was in a very rebellious mood. There was a circular newly laid flower bed creating a roundabout in front of the Trust headquarters, filled with cheerful scarlet poppies and looking absolutely beautiful. As I approached it for the last time I stopped and looked at it. For a moment, I was tempted to plough straight through it. But of course I didn't, that would be wanton, reckless damage, which isn't my style.

Instead, as I drove past each security camera en route to the gate I held up my middle finger, waving it aloft outside the window of my car. If I'd have been able to flash some offensive part of my anatomy and still drive in a straight line I might have done that too.

It was childish, but satisfying all the same.

Now I'm acting out, I thought, *analyse that!* My small act of defiance was one of the many similar, silent acts that took place daily in that dysfunctional institution. It's the kind of thing people do when they are disaffected, feeling that they aren't valued or listened to. As Martin Luther King said, 'A riot is the language of the unheard.' Looking back, it seems to me that for a long time a hushed, slow-motion sort of riot had been taking place.

*

A year on from leaving my hospital post, I received an almost carbon-copy request from Clifford's solicitor, asking me to carry out another memory assessment of his client. Clifford faced two more shoplifting charges and was once more using the defence that he 'forgot to pay'. Like Groundhog Day, I was instructed to confine my report to a description of his memory functioning and I was informed up front that Clifford would not allow me to request his medical files from his GP. Now I was the one sighing wearily.

My shoulders slumped a little when Clifford arrived at the solicitor's office wearing the same raincoat over another pair of oversized trousers and with a fresh batch of photocopied correspondence in his groaning satchel.

'Hello, I'm Clifford, not Cliff.'

'Hello, Clifford. We've met before, do you remember? My name's Kerry.' It seemed worth a try.

'Of course you are. I'm terrible with faces but I never forget names, Katie.'

Frustratingly for both of us, Groundhog Day it was, with Clifford once again struggling to fill in the blanks in his past and derailing my prompting by producing reams of letters he'd written to 'the authorities', 'the State' and the 'supposedly "Great" British Justice System'.

I repeated the WMS-III, the results of which were consistent with his previous year's scores. *At least there has been no deterioration*, I thought. Given the precedent set, my report might well be enough to get him off his latest set of charges. Another triumph for Clifford but not for the justice system.

Clifford's case was sticking in my craw. At the end of our meeting, he put back his shoulders and puffed out his chest so much that some of the creases in his shirt disappeared. 'We're fighting the system, you and me,' he declared, before adding, 'and we're winning, aren't we?' With that he gave me a conspiratorial wink.

And 'we' did go on to win again, in court at least. And again. And again. Clifford was referred to me nearly every year for five more years, at the end of which he was about to enter his sixth decade, but looked much older.

Every time his solicitor called, part of me wanted to say, 'Stop! Enough's enough! I'm not doing this again!' But who was I to take the moral high ground? Clifford was entitled to defend himself and I was hardly irreplaceable. If I didn't do the assessment, Clifford's solicitor would simply ask another psychologist to take on the work. Besides, I had added in some other psychometrics and was building up a nice little store of test results that I hoped, in vain, he might one day allow me to share with his doctor.

On the last occasion I saw him, the office in the precinct was occupied so I was invited to carry out my assessment at Clifford's flat. I didn't mind the change of scene, even when the first thing I saw when I arrived at his block of flats was a graffitied, ejaculating penis daubed on the wall in green paint. It was the only splash of colour in an otherwise concrete jungle, but at least this felt less like déjà vu.

'Good to see you, Katie,' Clifford boomed as he answered the door.

I told him it was good to see him again too, because, even though he was undeniably a user and abuser of my services, I still had a soft spot for him. I would have liked to tell him he looked well but it wasn't true. Clifford looked more crumpled and careworn than before, and a little more fragile.

His flat was tiny but fastidiously tidy. There was a postage stamp-sized kitchen, a living area with a sofa and a perfectly made-up mattress on the floor, and a box room, which he said he'd chosen to use as an office instead of a bedroom.

'It's where I write my letters and job-application forms, you see. Often I'm so exhausted from working that when I come out of the office to make a cup of tea I'm grateful to see my mattress there. Sometimes when I lie down I'm so very tired I stay there for a couple of days.'

I was sensing an air of defeat around Clifford, like he was struggling to keep on fighting, though who wouldn't be tired after more than 20 years of unemployment, disappointment and rejection?

We went through the motions of the assessment. Absolutely nothing had changed and all of Clifford's test results remained static. For a minute or two we sat in silence, like a pair of deflating balloons. I think we both felt equally demoralized, but Clifford suddenly cut through the cloud of melancholy that had descended. 'Come into my office,' he said perkily, getting to his feet. 'I want to show you some of my letters I've been writing.'

Here we go again, I thought.

I followed him into the little box room where something

immediately caught my eye. There on the wall above the desk was a framed degree certificate from Manchester University. Next to it was a certificate from a London college of further education. I studied both with great interest. Clifford M Booth had indeed gained a diploma in social policy in 1980 and a first-class degree in sociology in 1983. Beside the certificates were pictures of a clean-shaven, ironed young Clifford in a gown and mortarboard, beaming proudly for the camera.

'Look at you!' I said.

He nodded. 'I told you I was a socialist, didn't I? There's the proof, right there.' He pointed to another photograph, showing him smiling broadly, in line at what looked like a march. He was holding up a *Socialist Worker* placard that said 'Victory to the Miners'.

'You look happy, and handsome too, I must say.'

'My mum always says I could have had the pick of the girls when I was a young man,' he nodded, preening his shock of greying hair.

'Was there anyone special?' I asked.

Clifford thought about this very carefully and took his time in answering me.

'Yes,' he said eventually. 'There was somebody. It didn't work out but I can't remember a lot about her. My mum says I was never the same after we broke up.'

'In what way?'

Clifford said he didn't really know but his mother maintained that he'd 'had a nervous breakdown'.

This was new information, even though I'd asked numerous questions about his mental health in a variety of different ways over the years.

'You know, Clifford, I understand how you feel about your medical records but I still feel that it would be very helpful to me, and more importantly for you, if I could take a look. Because there might be some information in there that might help me to better understand the problems you have with your memory. It would only be me who sees them.' I didn't want to set him on another rant about human rights but at this juncture it felt like my professional duty to push for this.

Whether it was the intimacy of the setting or whether, after all these years, Clifford felt he could finally trust me, he agreed. 'OK, then,' he sighed. 'If you insist.'

Clifford signed the consent form and I explained that it would take a few weeks for the records to be released from his GP via his solicitor.

'Right you are, Katie.'

As I drove away, the ejaculating penis shrinking in my rear-view mirror, an indescribable wave of helplessness washed over me. Instead of having to write yet another report for the courts, I wished I had it in my power to prescribe Clifford a mission, a role in life with a sense of acceptance and validation. I'd seen the proof that as a young man, Clifford had been an impressive scholar and had good prospects. I'm sure he had been taken seriously. What had happened to him around the time of his 'nervous breakdown'? Was it responsible for leaving him clutching at the threads of his past? And stealing ridiculous items just for the novel high of believing he'd made an impact on the world?

I felt a buzz of excitement when Clifford's medical records arrived in the post. They might not tell me anything but I still felt as though I'd achieved something just by getting my hands on them. The mix of handwritten doctors' notes and typed letters looked disappointingly thin but I poured myself a cup of tea before sitting down to read them.

The notes went back as far as Clifford's early teens. He'd suffered from routine stomach upsets and ear infections, nothing out of the ordinary. During his university years, he fractured a bone in his shin while coaching a youth football team, so not only had Clifford once been an academic but he was a fit and sporty young man, an active member of the community. It was hard to reconcile the figure he had become with the dynamic 20-something he'd once been.

In his early twenties, Clifford had visited his GP in a 'distressed state'. By then, he was studying for a postgraduate social-work certificate and he told the doctor his girlfriend had broken off their relationship and he was finding it hard to cope. A month later, he was admitted to a psychiatric hospital where he was observed to be 'almost catatonic', lying motionless in bed, only sporadically interacting with nursing staff to tell them that his life no longer felt worth living.

Over a four-week period, Clifford was given eight sessions of ECT – electroconvulsive therapy – sometimes known as 'electric shock treatment'.

My jaw fell open as the penny dropped. I thought of the

infamous scene in *One Flew Over the Cuckoo's Nest,* where Jack Nicholson's wayward character, pinned to a bed by four orderlies, is given the procedure as a punishment and without general anaesthetic.

I knew relatively little about ECT, other than that it was a subject guaranteed to cause passionate debate, if not out-and-out war, in a room of psychologists and psychiatrists.

It started out as a controversial experiment in the 1930s when psychiatrists noticed that the mood of distressed patients seemed to lift following an epileptic fit. In order to create the same effect artificially, they placed electrodes on the scalps of patients diagnosed with depression or expressing suicidal intent, applying 150 volts of electric current – enough to induce a seizure in the brain. With no real understanding of how it might work, as well as being used as a treatment for low mood and depression, until the 1950s ECT was also given as a supposed 'cure' for homosexuality.

Early anecdotes exist of nurses having to chase petrified patients around ECT suites, though thankfully it hasn't been given without anaesthesia for many decades. I've never seen it being carried out but over the years I've consoled nurses who've been sickened by witnessing their charges' hands and feet jerking and twitching as they 'fit'. When the patients start to wake up and the nurse brings them tea and a slice of toast, the question they most often ask is, 'Where am I?'

Still, around 2,500 patients in the UK have ECT every year, most commonly older women who, like the late Carrie Fisher, believe it might help improve their mood. 'Over time, this fucking thing punched the dark lights out of my depression,' Fisher wrote in her 2011 memoir, *Shockaholic*. 'It was like a mute button muffling the noise of my shrieking feelings.' She admitted that her memory was damaged by ECT – a documented side-effect – but in her experience, it was worth the loss. Not so for Ernest Hemingway, who found the memory loss devastating. 'What is the sense of ruining my head and erasing my memory, which is my business?' he said, famously adding, 'It was a brilliant cure, but we lost the patient.' Hemingway killed himself in 1961, shortly after having 20 rounds of ECT.

John Read, professor of clinical psychology at the University of East London, is a long-term critic of what many – myself now included – consider an archaic practice. In 2013, he argued that, rather than addressing the causes of depression, ECT systematically and gradually wipes out patients' memory and cognitive functions. 'I'm convinced that in 10 or 15 years we will have put electroconvulsive therapy in the same rubbish bin of historical treatments as lobotomies and surprise [ice] baths that have been discarded over time,' he stated.

Read went on to conduct a major review of ECT research literature with Professor Irving Kirsch of Harvard Medical School, published in June 2020 in the *Journal of Ethical Human Psychology and Psychiatry*. It found 'very little evidence' that ECT was any better than placebo in the short-term and 'no evidence at all beyond the end of treatment'. The review concluded that there was also no evidence that ECT saves lives by preventing suicide, as its supporters often claim. 'On the other side of the cost-benefit equation,' it went on, 'there is a slight but significant risk of death, and between 12 and 55 percent of ECT recipients suffer brain damage in the form of permanent memory loss.'

Incidentally, the 12 to 55 per cent seems to differ depending on who you ask – the treating psychiatrists or their patients.

Unsettling as this was, Clifford's memory problems now made sense. According to a second discharge summary, his mood briefly picked up following the ECT but he was admitted to hospital again, complaining of amnesia and suddenly being unable to read. He was disabled by fatigue, saying it felt like his mind was 'closing down'. Clifford was diagnosed with a relapse of his 'depressive disorder'. He was prescribed a second round of ECT, making 16 sessions in total, and this is where his hospital notes ran out.

I was left wondering, who are we, without our memories? The man I was working with had an irrepressible spirit but he was stitched together from a few old photographs, mementos and anecdotes told by his mother. It wasn't just his memories that had been destroyed: so much of Clifford's potential had been lost, too. He'd had his heart broken, yet psychiatry's response had been to attach him to the mains supply and damage his brain, leaving him a remnant of the person he once was.

I held off writing my report until I'd told Clifford what I had found. Sitting in his box-room office, he looked absolutely surprised and told me he couldn't remember having the treatment.

'Do you recall it ever being discussed with you?' I ventured. Nowhere in his meagre medical record could I find any evidence that the risks of ECT had been explained to him, or that he'd even consented to have it. As he shrugged his shoulders, I wondered if, at the time, he might have gambled on forgetting the pain of a lost romance. I couldn't imagine him in any way comprehending the harm that was about to be inflicted on him.

'I don't want to jump to any conclusions,' I said delicately, 'but I wonder if the ECT is connected to your amnesia and the problems you have taking in new information. I'd love to send a note to your GP with the results of the assessments we've done. I think it would be helpful to add them to your notes and perhaps it would be useful for you to see a neuropsychologist who would be able to interpret them much better than I can.'

'No,' he said cheerily. 'I'm going to get a job soon so I will be too busy. Everything is going well. We're fighting persecution by the nitwits in our so-called justice system, you and me. And look, I got one of my letters published in the *Bolton Evening News*.'

He showed me a letter, which looked like so many others I'd seen before, protesting against an increase in bus fares, council tax or the price of the Lord Mayor's dry cleaning.

I took a deep breath, wondering how I could get through to him.

'Please listen to me, Clifford. I am not going to carry on writing reports for you. Shoplifting costs UK retailers over a billion pounds each year. The cost to the shops is passed on to the customers – customers like you and me.'

Clifford opened his mouth to object but I held my hand up. 'Don't tell me that you forgot to pay because I don't believe you.' I said firmly. 'This time you had three blocks of Stilton round one ankle and two cans of shaving foam round the other. Shoplifting is *anti*social, not a socialist thing to do at all. You need to stop. You are a man of the people and you need to look after your fellow citizens, not put their shopping bills up.'

Clifford nodded petulantly. Perhaps we had finally reached an understanding. As we parted ways, I wished him luck and repeated that I hoped never to see him under these circumstances again. This time I finally got my wish. Whether he gave up his light-fingered protests or just stopped getting caught, Clifford was never referred to me again.

He was not the model citizen he could and should have been but I still think of him fondly. A misfit of psychiatry's making, he had become a shrewd player of our legal system, capitalizing on memory problems that had nothing directly to do with his petty shoplifting and yet everything to do with it. I'm unlikely to forget him. And I am unlikely to forgive what was stolen from him, in the name of mental-health treatment.

CHAPTER THREE
IN LIES, TRUTH

I watched, transfixed, as the baby's arm stiffened and outstretched, his head turned to the side and his eyes and mouth opened wide, like a soprano reaching for the last, highest note.

The staff darted in all directions. A support worker was on her knees, calmly moving away brightly coloured plastic blocks, soft books with tiny mirrors and plastic teething rings attached to them and, surprisingly, a pink fabric pig wearing a crinkly red dress. As she picked it up the pig announced, 'I'm so pretty...oink!', the surrealness of which snapped my attention back to the room.

'Let's all take a break and make some space,' I said to anyone still listening. An underwhelming contribution, but this was not a situation that I'd planned for in the middle of delivering a staff training session in the mural-covered lounge of a mother-and-baby unit. The pebble-dashed, two-storey building was one of two butted together in an area where businesses leaking out of Liverpool city centre met 1970s residential housing. The facility contained one-bedroom flats for up to 12 mums and their babies or young children, and occasionally their partners.

I suddenly felt pretty useless. I've never considered myself the maternal type – if I ever told my friends that I was eating for two, they'd think I'd got a tapeworm – but seeing this 11-month-old baby fitting and not being able to do anything to help him was making my throat feel numb and my eyes sting. I watched in admiration as the unruffled support worker gently placed two cushions either side of the baby's body to keep him as safe as possible while the seizure burned itself out. 'There we are, Callum,' she soothed.

He was red in the face and his pudgy legs were jerking, pulling his knees up to his stomach. The support worker reached down and loosened the poppers at the neck of his baby-gro.

Most of the staff had dispersed by now but I stayed put, not having anywhere else to go.

The room smelt of soap and that chemical lemony scent of baby wipes. It's a smell I associate with having car sickness as a child, one that still makes me feel slightly nauseous as I'm reminded of Mum mopping me up while my stomach and head swam in opposite directions.

I sat in silence as Callum's limbs finally stilled and the support worker expertly scooped him up into the baby recovery position, cradling him in her arms with his head tilted downwards.

'Shall I take him?' I heard someone say.

I turned to see an elfin-like woman rushing into the room. She was dressed in pyjamas and a silk dressing gown and had a baby-changing bag over her shoulder that seemed almost as big as she was. 'I've been shown how to do that at the hospital,' she offered, her voice loaded with concern.

Before the support worker could reply, two paramedics dashed in, manoeuvring their bulky equipment between the armchairs.

'Are you Mum?' one of them asked.

'Yes, I'm Adele. He's my son. Is he OK? He hasn't been well for months....' The support worker handed Callum to the medics and put her arm around the mother. 'He's been seeing a paediatric neurologist,' Adele offered.

As the paramedics got to work, she began relaying the little boy's extensive medical history in a succinct and impressively knowledgeable manner. Staff at the unit had just been telling me about Adele, describing her as polite, cooperative and appreciative of their help. I certainly saw this for myself as she talked to the paramedics.

'Please, I think my baby needs to be checked out at the hospital, thank you. Can I come in the ambulance with my son, please? Oh, you've been wonderful with my son, I'm so grateful.'

My son. I noticed that Adele didn't once refer to Callum by name.

Minutes later, I was alone, listening to the sound of the siren disappearing outside, hoping the baby would be OK.

I thought back over what else I'd been told about Adele. I'd been in the middle of delivering a safeguarding training session, detailing what the staff at the unit needed to do to ensure that none of their residents were exposed to harm, when I was told that Callum was joining us while his mum had a break. A baby in the room isn't ideal but you have to improvise in all manner of situations when asked to deliver training on site. The little boy grizzled and cried whether he was being carried, put down or rocked in a bouncy cradle chair, and none of the toys interested him. When his cries escalated to raucous wails that were drowning me out, the support worker had taken him outside for a while.

Before I could resume the training session, the staff had taken full advantage of the interruption and began telling me all about Adele. She was clearly a character who'd caught their attention – and divided opinion – because an animated group conversation ensued.

'She's such a lovely girl and a really good mum, such a shame she's had to go through all this.'

'So polite. A breath of fresh air.'

'I'm not so sure. I'd trust her a bit more if she gave us a hard time like the rest of 'em!'

'How can you say that? It must be horrendous for a mother to be accused of something like that, she must be petrified of putting a foot wrong.'

'You know what they say, no smoke without fire…'

Adele was under suspicion of harming Callum and had come willingly to the unit to allow social services to closely monitor both her and her son's progress. I was told the 21-year-old had been part way through a university degree when she fell pregnant. Her boyfriend, a fellow student, told her he didn't want to be a father and, after completing her second year, she left university and returned to her family home to have the baby.

Callum had a history of stopping breathing and going limp. Adele had performed CPR and revived him several times, both at home and in hospital, but medics had become suspicious because she was always on her own with her baby when he stopped breathing.

The staff at the mother-and-baby unit were very experienced in dealing with mothers who injured their babies in a moment of stress or with rough, careless handling. They were also used to parents who lacked knowledge and understanding about how to care for their child. But a 'lovely', 'gentle' and 'educated' young mother accused of deviously and repeatedly harming her baby? Not so easy to compute.

In the last six weeks Callum had had two seizures, both witnessed by staff at the unit.

'The poor girl's had such a rough time of it,' one support worker said sympathetically. 'He's clearly a sickly baby, he has chronic constipation and rarely settles. Left on her own, she barely gets the chance to sleep or wash.'

That was why staff had taken the unusual step of giving Adele an hour and a half to herself every day.

In an effort to guide the conversation back to the topic in hand, I asked what the risk-management plan was for Callum when he and his mum arrived at the unit.

'They're in one of the flats with CCTV. Adele is monitored by a member of staff all the time she's with Callum. They're escorted in communal areas and whenever they have to leave the unit, to go to hospital, shopping and so on.'

'And when she's not with Callum?'

An awkward silence fell. I wasn't trying to be clever. That's how any forensic psychologist's mind would work, especially in the thick of a safeguarding session interrupted by a baby suspected of being deliberately harmed by his mother. Good risk management is all about crossing your t's and dotting your i's. There can be no margin for error because as middle class, well educated and 'lovely' as Adele may have been in the eyes of most of the staff, she was still under investigation for suspected child abuse. The stakes, for both her and her son, couldn't get much higher.

Three years previously, in 2007, I'd come to the same mother-and-baby unit to meet Justine, a young mum with a nine-week-old son called Jasper. I remembered the visit very well, not least because as I stood at the door, waiting to be let in, the cardboard tube of a toilet roll hit me on the top of the head. When I stepped backwards and looked up – probably not the most sensible thing to do when unexpected toilet-related objects are raining from above – I saw an angry-faced woman sitting astride the apex of the roof, toilet paper streamers running away from her in all directions, like white icing drizzled over the top of a cake. I'd heard of rooftop protests in prisons, but never in a mother-and-baby unit!

In most instances, the parents at the unit had been directed by the Family Courts or the local authority to complete a 12-week residential parenting programme. Staff were required to keep a detailed log for social workers or to present as evidence in court and in some cases, every single second a parent spent with their child had to be accounted for. Inevitably, it made for an intense and taxing dynamic. Pass muster and you got to leave and start a new life as an independent family unit. Fail and your baby might be taken away, either into long-term care or put up for adoption. The mothers were understandably stressed, emotionally charged and anxious. It was hardly surprising that a siege mentality sometimes set in.

'Oh, Justine! How did you get up there?' shouted the unit manager who had come to let me in. She was now frowning up at the rooftop protester.

Justine. She was the mother I'd come to see. One chance in 12 – it had to be my client, didn't it?

I knew Justine had recently turned 20 but she looked older, in a careworn way. Her skin was tired and dark around the eyes, her over-bleached hair scraped into a dull, lifeless ponytail.

'Get my social worker!' she yelled. 'I want my baby back! I'm staying here until you get my social worker.'

'This is the psychologist who's come to see you,' the unit manager called back, to which Justine responded by launching another toilet roll missile.

As it landed at my feet she shouted, 'You don't fucking know me! Who do you think you are? You're like some fucking judge who doesn't know me and has taken my baby off me. I want to see my social worker, not a fucking psychologist!'

I was confused because I'd been told that Justine was doing well with Jasper and embracing the support she was receiving at the unit. When I asked the manager what had gone on, she let out a long sigh.

'She'd been getting on so well but Jasper had to be taken into foster care this morning.'

Justine's key worker, the person who worked most closely with her, joined us outside. She was another mature and no-nonsense type of woman, dressed in baggy jeans and a mohair cardigan. Between us we managed to convince Justine to come down and show me the photos of Jasper she kept in her flat. Once she'd finally agreed, she slid five foot down the terracotta tiles and dropped like a stone onto the rusty fire escape at the side. She made her descent look easy, though I still held my breath as I watched her.

As we walked to her flat Justine wouldn't speak to me or her key worker, or even make eye contact. But by the time we were in her living room and I'd seen several pictures of her saucer-eyed baby boy, she was crying like a toddler, snot and tears bubbling from her face as she curled herself into a ball on her stiff little sofa.

'I always mess it up. Was I born wrong? I didn't mean it. I just needed a break. Will I get Jasper back? Can I have him back?'

The long and short of it was that Justine had asked if she could go to the local shop a few days earlier, leaving Jasper with the staff for 'half an hour'. When she was out, she bought and ate a packet of crab sticks, knowing full well that she was dangerously allergic to shellfish.

'Things could have turned out very differently,' the unit manager said, explaining that when Justine finally got herself to A&E her skin had broken out in red blotches and her throat was so swollen she was fighting to breathe. 'She went into anaphylactic shock. If she wasn't trying to kill herself, she very nearly did.'

It was impossible to give Justine any reassurances about getting her son back. It wasn't simply the concern she'd caused by deliberately threatening her own life, the reason she was on social services' radar in the first place was that she'd already had one child taken off her – a daughter, Lacey, who was found with unexplained injuries. Justine had a lot to prove. And to make matters worse, the political wind was not blowing in her favour.

Peter Connelly – the 17-month-old known as 'Baby P' – had been killed in August of the same year. A post-mortem examination found that he had over 50 separate injuries, including a broken back and ribs, that had been caused or allowed by his mother, her boyfriend and his brother over an eight-month period. Peter had been well known to Haringey social services and the NHS. A serious case review was initiated as press and politicians demanded to know why he hadn't been protected by them.

The fear of having one's head on the chopping block in the event of 'another Baby P' is thought to have contributed to the highly risk-averse culture that had begun to permeate children's services. Office for National Statistics (ONS) data show a rapid increase in the number of babies removed from their mothers at birth after Peter's death, with cases more than doubling between 2008 and 2013, from 802 to 2,018.

I'd been brought in at the request of the Family Court to carry out a psychological assessment of Justine, but rather than put her through any additional torment that day I left her, quiet and exhausted, rocked in the woolly arms of her key worker.

I saw Justine the following week, still without Jasper and in the emergency accommodation she'd been moved to. Her paperwork had made dispiriting reading and today she looked subdued, far less animated than she had been when she was furious on the roof.

It's a sad fact that Justine's background was fairly typical of a lot of young women I'd encountered going through legal proceedings in the hope of being able to keep their children. Raised in poverty, she had no idea who her father was and, according to one social-services report, neighbours described her mother as more interested in 'gallivanting, drinking, drugs, partying, having new boyfriends and new babies' than looking after Justine and her younger siblings. The children were left alone at night while their mother went out and, depending on her mood when she came home, Justine might be dragged out of bed by her hair as a punishment for being 'lazy' and not cleaning the house.

When she was 12, Justine spent 18 months in foster care, the only period of her childhood she remembered with any fondness. She recalled 'being on a beach and going on holiday to London'. Poignantly, she also said, 'My breakfast was done for me....I was told to go to bed and I felt loved and cared for.' Those last details jumped off the page and I felt a pang of sympathy. A breakfast, a set bedtime and feeling loved and cared for. Basic needs for any child and things I'd taken for granted in my own comfortable childhood. I'd have been baffled if another child had told me they actually *wanted* a set bedtime. The lucky ones among us only ever saw the injustice of being sent to bed before the 9pm watershed.

Reading Justine's notes, I felt acutely grateful not only for the upbringing I'd had but for the life I was leading. Going into full-time private practice had been one of my better decisions and, over the last four years, a rich variety of work had flowed in. I loved being my own boss, writing up psychology reports from home in my onesie, though I did find that I missed the day-to-day interactions with my psychology and nursing teams (and my patients) that had been part of hospital life. At one hospital I'd worked at, we kept a honking rubber chicken in the staff room that we would squeeze – staff and patients alike – when we felt like screaming. A honk from the chicken was the signal that someone needed a listening ear, a pep-talk or maybe just a cup of tea and some quiet company. I'd learned that nothing compares to the immediate informal debriefing and support you receive from the colleagues you work with day in, day out.

Working independently, I still had monthly supervision meetings with another psychologist but that scheduled hour with an agenda to get through, although essential, just doesn't feel the same. It meant that after a couple of years of being a one-woman band, I'd branched out to run a small but busy team of psychologists and psychotherapists working across the north of England. Advising in Family Court cases was not an area I'd ever envisaged working in but as my reputation within the criminal courts grew, so too did requests to work with clients like Justine.

Justine didn't finish her education, let alone enjoy the luxury of choosing a career. With 'limited literacy skills' because of her repeated absences from school, she had stopped attending altogether at 14 and started working in a takeaway. A few days short of her sixteenth birthday, in walked a 27-year-old man who 'flattered' her with his attention. Within weeks, he had asked her to move in with him and their daughter Lacey was born ten months later.

When the baby was eight months old, Justine pulled back the cover in her cot and found the little girl blue around the mouth and with blood dripping from her nose.

'Help me, please!' Justine screamed when she called 999 in a frantic panic. 'My baby's bleeding! There's something wrong with her! Please come quickly!'

Lacey was rushed to Alder Hey Children's Hospital, where the community paediatrician found bruises on both sides of her face. Neither parent could account for the injuries, though the doctor concluded they were consistent with the child having been slapped or punched. Justine was fiercely adamant she had never laid a finger on her baby, but so too was Lacey's father. Despite their pleas and Justine's increasingly angry protests, social services were called and Lacey swiftly became the subject of care proceedings. After a multitude of assessments, the judge concluded that the little girl would be at risk of significant harm if she were to return to either parent. By the time Lacey had turned two, she had become one of the small number of children in care to find a new, permanent adoptive family.

Justine's more recent notes told me that during her pregnancy with Jasper – whose father was listed as 'unknown' – she had been in and out of hospital complaining of collapsing, blood loss and sickness, though multiple tests and investigations had failed to find the cause. The last time she was admitted, a nurse pulled back the blue curtain around her bed to find her adding packets of salt to a plastic jug of water. Justine also had a half-empty packet of laxatives, cementing suspicions that she was deliberately trying to induce vomiting and diarrhoea.

'You interfering bitch!' she'd screamed when the nurse confronted her.

As is usual in family-law cases, I'd been given a long list of questions, approved by all parties in the case, to cover in my assessment. The overall purpose was to assess Justine's 'level of insight into Jasper's physical and emotional needs for security, stability and appropriate protection' and her 'ability to meet those needs and prioritize them over her own'. In short, was she capable of being a good enough parent?

Having been through what must be this incredibly invasive process before, Justine fully understood that my opinion could help make or break her reunion with Jasper and, though she looked uncomfortable when I first arrived, hugging herself defensively against the back of an armchair, she opened a packet of biscuits and did her best to cooperate.

She told me that Lacey's dad had started hitting her and locking her in the house when she fell pregnant. He didn't want anyone 'asking questions' (while their 'relationship' wasn't strictly illegal, it was more than a little morally dubious), so she wasn't even allowed to go to the GP. The result was that she gave birth at home, alone.

'It was after I had Lacey he started getting even more angry with me. One night we argued. A really bad argument. He punched me in the face and…'

Her top lip was wobbling. She bit on it and I saw that her teeth were grey and crumbling. Poverty and neglect leave a multitude of legacies, I thought, not all so depressingly obvious.

'What happened after he hit you?'

'I just wanted it to stop, I just needed to get away. I was panicking so I pretended to faint. He stopped hitting me then. He was nice to me after, said he was sorry, made me a brew.'

After Lacey 'got hurt' and social services got involved, Justine's partner became all the more controlling, she said. One night, after she'd chewed the inside of her mouth in anxiety and spat out a thick glob of blood, he reluctantly 'allowed' her to go to the hospital. 'He only let me because I pretended I was coughing up blood. I kept up the lie when I got to hospital but I told the nurse when he wasn't there that I didn't want to go back home.'

It was then that she disclosed for the first time that her partner had been violent towards their baby, too. Justine was moved to a women's refuge. At that point in the proceedings, a reunion with Lacey was not entirely out of the question. Justine was in the midst of a full schedule of parenting assessments and supervised contact visits, and no decision had yet been made about her daughter's long-term future. But then she suddenly stopped attending the sessions, telling social workers she was 'too ill', effectively putting the first drops of ink on Lacey's adoption papers.

'It's not that I didn't love her, you know,' she said, gnawing her lip again. 'I don't know...sometimes I thought I must just be a bad mum and she would be better off without me.'

I started to push her about her recent hospital visits, treading an invisible tightrope in attempting not to imply I was judging her but being clear that I knew she had been found with the salt and the laxatives. The questions still rattled her. She looked ashamed, a red flush creeping from the edge of her round-necked jumper and flaring across her neck.

'I don't like being sick, I actually hate being sick,' she insisted, her voice rising. 'And I wasn't trying to kill myself eating those crab sticks, you know. I made a mistake. I forgot.'

I didn't believe for a minute that Justine had forgotten she was allergic to shellfish but I did believe the rest of it. There was an obvious pattern here, with fabricated and induced illnesses becoming reliable friends to Justine in her lowest moments. As unpleasant as it was to feel ill, it was a price she was willing to pay when she hit the threshold of her ability to cope. Her medical records showed that while she'd been in and out of A&E complaining of unexplained maladies, hospital staff had noticed that she seemed desperate to be admitted and stay as long as possible. Who could blame her? The respite and care she received when she assumed the role of a patient was unavailable anywhere else in her life.

We all need TLC at times. When I was about seven and fancied a day or two with a blanket on the sofa watching *Pipkins* and *Pebble Mill* (God, I'm so old), I made my own vomit out of porridge oats and poured it in the loo. Then I started retching dramatically until my mum came to my aid and popped a thermometer in my mouth. As soon as she left the room, I pulled it out and stuck it in my hot-water bottle cover. When Mum returned, the toasty thermometer was back under my tongue and I was doing my best impression of a dying swan. It was all going so well, until later in the day when I made the mistake of holding the thermometer in front of the fire to show Mum *exactly* how feverish I was. The mercury couldn't cope and the thermometer exploded in my hand. That was it. Me and the thermometer were both busted. But nearly 40 years on, if I've got a cold and feel sorry for myself, I'll still go to my mum's house and croak pathetically on her sofa in the hope of a bit of chicken soup and sympathy.

'By playing sick, we gained sympathy, care, and attention, and were excused from our responsibilities' note Marc Feldman and Gregory Yates in *Dying to Be Ill,* a study of the lived experience of those who feign sickness. 'Though doing so on occasion is considered normal,' the authors continue, 'there are those who carry their deceptions to the extreme.'

In extreme circumstances, Justine had learned to become an extreme medical deceiver.

When it came to writing up my findings for the court (still at home and in my onesie), the Philip Larkin poem 'This Be the Verse' ran through my head. In it, he describes the ever-deepening misery that is handed down from generation to generation, unless you heed his advice to 'get out as early as you can'.

Justine had been damaged and made vulnerable by the miserable, neglected upbringing she had suffered and abuse at the hands of the adults she relied upon. In many ways, she'd done an incredible job with Jasper but in care proceedings the focus is not on what a parent has achieved despite the odds, or indeed on how they will feel if their child is removed from them – the welfare of the child trumps everything. My job was to work through my list of questions with a beady, unblinking eye on Jasper's needs and future wellbeing, and that alone.

Writing up my report was not a pleasant task. I would have needed to be carved from marble not to appreciate the impact it would have on Justine if she lost her second child, but she was not equipped to meet his needs. As I typed my final sentence it felt like I was hanging a heavy weight around the neck of an already drowning girl.

*

I hadn't expected to ever see Adele again but later in 2010, ten weeks after Callum's admission to hospital, we were sitting opposite each other in a dimly lit room, in stony-faced silence.

Tests had revealed high quantities of over-the-counter antihistamines in Callum's bloodstream. A review of the CCTV footage taken when Adele had been alone in her flat at the mother-and-baby unit showed her adding bottles of liquid antihistamine syrup to her son's meals on two separate occasions. She was later filmed hurriedly emptying her fridge of the little plastic food containers, swilling their incriminating contents down the sink.

When confronted, Adele eventually admitted her guilt and was remanded in prison, awaiting sentencing for two counts of child cruelty. Her mother had immediately leapt into action, enlisting the services of a flashy London legal firm and paying for an opinion from a private psychiatrist.

The psychiatrist must have been old school because he'd diagnosed Adele with 'Munchausen syndrome by proxy', which by 2010 was a tarnished and outdated label, albeit one still trotted out today. The peculiarity of the name, and its quirky origin, have undoubtedly contributed to its staying power.

Baron Munchausen is a fictional character inspired by a real-life 18th-century nobleman who was famous not for feigning illness but for entertaining his upper-crust friends with exaggerated tales about his military career. The German writer Rudolf Erich Raspe adapted the tall tales into his 1785 novel *Baron Munchausen's Narrative of His Marvellous*

Travels and Campaigns in Russia, playing on the nobleman's catalogue of fantastical claims, such as riding on a cannonball and fighting a 40-foot crocodile.

Fast-forward to 1951 and the term 'Munchausen syndrome' was coined by Richard Asher, a physician known for his provocative writing. In an article in *The Lancet*, he described three cases of patients presenting themselves at hospital after hospital in severe abdominal pain, having coughed up pints of blood. Each had a 'gridiron stomach', Asher's way of illustrating the criss-cross of livid white scars on their skin from multiple emergency surgeries. The trio had something else in common, too: their complaints were all entirely false.

'Like the famous Baron von Munchausen, the persons affected have always travelled widely; and their stories, like those attributed to him, are both dramatic and untruthful,' Asher wrote.

Once Asher's baby had been christened with its flamboyant name, the medical congregation rushed to embrace it. The article released a flood of similar reports from doctors describing patients – often quite ingeniously – fabricating everything from urinary-tract infections to leukaemia and psychological trauma, all seemingly in the hope of garnering the sympathy and attention associated with assuming the sick role.

A second variation of the syndrome was proposed in 1976, when the term 'Munchausen syndrome by proxy' (MSbP) first appeared in a paper by New Zealand psychologists

John Money and June Faith Werlwas. It was subsequently popularized by the highly publicized work of British paediatrician Professor Roy Meadow. In a series of influential papers, Meadow detailed the cases of six-year-old Kay and fourteen-month-old Charles whose mothers, he claimed, had knowingly sabotaged their children's health for perverse emotional reward. Their methods were quite different – one used her own blood to contaminate urine samples, the other poisoned her child repeatedly with salt – but their attitudes and behaviour were strikingly similar. He noted that both parents had faked illness before becoming parents, had 'an insatiable appetite for good paediatric units, staffed with sympathetic doctors and nurses... [and received] gratification from the child's illness upon their own life'.

Meadow was at pains to point out that the goal of his work was to improve the recognition and management of a specific form of child abuse, rather than to encourage the 'MSbP' label to be applied to perpetrators. It therefore came as a thunderbolt to many that he went on to support the inclusion of 'MSbP' in the *Diagnostic and Statistical Manual of Mental Disorders*, albeit under a new brand. Since the publication of the third edition of the *Big Book of Human Suffering* in 1980, any blatant porky pie-telling or contrivances to fake ailments in yourself have been officially known as 'factitious disorder'. These days, 'factitious disorder imposed on another (FDIA)' is the preferred (and considerably less sexy) term for 'MSbP', though use of the latter persists, particularly in the media and the minds of the public. How ironic that 'the falsification of physical or psychological signs or symptoms, or induction of injury or disease, associated with identified deception' came to be considered a *genuine* mental 'illness' – by some, at least.

It isn't just parents who have the opportunity to medically abuse children. Meadow gave his 'expert' evidence in the case of Beverley Allitt, the 29-year-old nurse who murdered four children, attempted to kill three others and caused grievous bodily harm to six more on the children's ward at Grantham and Kesteven Hospital in Lincolnshire. Though police never discovered how she carried out all of her assaults, Allitt is believed to have suffocated some of her victims and injected air or large doses of drugs into others.

Allitt was convicted in 1993, but arguments regarding her mental state at the time of the killings, and the most appropriate sentencing option, rumbled on until 2007. Professor Meadow's opinion was that her offences were 'a most extreme case' of 'MSbP'. She was unlikely to have derived any pleasure from her criminal acts, he said, as her primary purpose was to draw attention to herself rather than to kill or injure children. Others strongly disagreed, pointing to the fact that Meadow was a paediatrician, not a forensic psychiatrist, and he had failed to grasp Allitt's history of sadistic behaviours. Dr Hamilton – Allitt's treating psychiatrist at Rampton Hospital, where she had been transferred from HMP Holloway upon refusing to eat or drink – sensibly informed the High Court of Justice that, in his view, Munchausen syndrome by proxy 'is not a mental disorder in its own right but is a complex of behaviours, habits and perhaps attitudes' stemming from both a seriously damaged personality and the life experiences and environment 'sufferers' find themselves in.

The judge agreed, commenting that 'to give a pattern of criminal behaviour a name does not of itself lessen the responsibility of the offender. One could say that a multiple rapist exhibits multiple rape syndrome but that would not of itself lessen his criminal responsibility and should not of itself lead to a lesser sentence.'

While he accepted that Allitt had a longstanding 'constellation of personality disorders', the judge upheld her original 13 concurrent terms of life imprisonment with a minimum 30-year tariff.

It would take a dozen years for Meadow's credibility – and, by association, the credibility of MSbP – to be comprehensively challenged. In the meantime, he went on to provide testimony in a string of cases involving mothers of children who had suffered cot deaths, including that of solicitor Sally Clark. His erroneous claim that there was a '1 in 73 million chance' of two such deaths occurring in families like the Clarks led to her wrongful conviction for murdering her two baby sons. During a fitness-to-practice hearing before the General Medical Council, Meadow apologized for the effect of his 'misleading' evidence. It was too late for Sally Clark, the effects of bereavement, the miscarriage of justice and her incarceration having taken an overwhelming toll. She died in 2007, as a result of acute alcohol intoxication.

*

I met Adele in a room reserved for legal meetings. One bald, dull lightbulb made the small interview space feel like a basement, though it was actually off to the side of the main prison visitors' area, which was filling up with people. As usual, all the inmates were wearing red sporty-type bibs to distinguish them from visitors, reminding me of a large netball team.

Adele's hair had been cut into a neat bob that suited her small, heart-shaped face. Quietly and politely, she thanked me for agreeing to provide a report for her sentence hearing as she took her seat across the laminate-topped table. She clasped her hands daintily in her lap, her shoulders drooping forward and her chin pointing at her collarbone, like Princess Diana outside the Taj Mahal. She seemed physically weighed down by guilt, or was it shame? Maybe she was simply embarrassed at having had the hypocrisy behind her diligent parent persona so nakedly revealed to me. Whatever it was, innate politeness seemed to be all that was propping her up.

Callum had had a precariously high heart rate when he arrived at hospital but had made a good recovery and was being cared for by Adele's mother. She had the support of social workers to apply to the Family Law Court for a Special Guardianship Order, allowing her to have long-term care of her grandson.

'I'm so grateful to my mother,' Adele said. 'I couldn't bear the idea of Callum being with strangers.'

Adele was the only child of wealthy parents who were both insurance brokers. Speaking very gently, she explained that their long hours meant they hadn't had much time to spend with her, the gaps being plugged by after-school clubs, Brownie camps and au pairs. Her parents went through a 'messy' divorce when she was eight, she said, her father moving out and maintaining contact via Christmas and birthday cards, sporadic cheques and increasingly infrequent phone calls.

'That's when my mother started working even longer hours. She made sure I had everything I wanted but we never had much fun together. She was a bit of a stranger, really.'

'How did you feel about that?'

There was no uncertainty in her answer. 'Lonely. Unimportant. And I was jealous of friends who had mothers that treated them like friends.'

When Adele fell pregnant and her boyfriend walked away from her, there was no question that she wouldn't keep the baby. 'I was excited to have someone that was going to be all mine, to love and care for,' she said dreamily, revealing more than she had intended.

The girls in her university flat rallied round to support her as she completed the second year of her music and history joint-honours degree. 'They helped me to do everything right. I was eating the right food, taking all the right supplements, exercising. They even took it in turns not to drink alcohol so that I didn't feel like the odd one out when we went out at night.'

I'd been surprised to find that Adele's medical records hadn't shown any suggestion of sham illnesses or seeking out medical attention. Although, as you would expect of most expectant mothers, she had been meticulous with her antenatal checks.

'Tell me about those,' I said.

A smile teased her lips. 'All the staff were so kind and mumsy. I got told off for riding a bike to my 20-week scan. I loved that!'

The remark took me back three years, to when I was carrying out my assessment of Justine for the Family Courts. 'I was told to go to bed and I felt loved and cared for.'

I remembered the effect Justine's words had on me, making me appreciate how much I'd taken for granted in my own childhood. I grew up in a working-class family in Manchester; my parents weren't wealthy but they were lavish with their love and care and generous with their time – intangible gifts it takes an adult eye to fully appreciate. Gifts that Adele, in spite of her otherwise privileged background, hadn't received.

After leaving university and returning home at seven months pregnant, Adele developed symphysis pubis dysfunction, a common but painful condition of pregnancy.

'Mum had retired by then. I had to use crutches to get around and she helped me a lot. She was great, actually, helping me with my physio. She suddenly couldn't do enough for me.'

'What did that feel like?'

'It was unexpected but I loved it. Mum told me she was proud of me for getting on with a difficult situation. She'd never said anything like that to me before. Even though I was in a lot of pain, I remember wishing that I could stay pregnant for longer.'

'That's quite a thing to say. How intense was the pain?'

'It was pretty bad,' she said, noncommittally.

'Were you ever tempted to exaggerate it or play on it in any way?'

'I might have exaggerated it a bit, you know...'

I nodded. 'I need you to fill these in as honestly as you possibly can,' I told her, patting a wad of questionnaires I'd brought along to get a measure of her personality. What I didn't tell her is that all the assessment tools I'd chosen had in-built validity scales that would pick up on whether or not she was able to be honest and open, or if she attempted to portray herself in a more positive (or negative) light than was realistic.

It took her an hour to fill them in. Each and every inventory showed that Adele had a definite bias towards presenting herself in a more socially desirable light than was likely to be the case (as maybe we all would if we knew a judge would soon be deciding our future). I adjusted her personality scales scores to compensate in the areas she hadn't been entirely honest and what emerged was a pattern of self-centredness mixed with crushingly low self-esteem. Those two traits may appear to contradict each other but, when you think about it, Adele had grown up in a contradictory environment, overindulged with material goods while simultaneously having her emotional needs overlooked. Sometimes, when you grow up feeling small and insignificant, you learn to compensate with selfishness.

With the psychometrics out of the way, it was time to get down to the nitty gritty.

Callum had been born at full term without any complications. Adele 'relished' being a mother, she told me. She 'loved Callum from the moment I laid eyes on him' and no, she insisted, her mood didn't drop in the months after his birth. She denied any thoughts about harming her child. So how, then, had she come to poison him?

Adele wasn't forthcoming with any answers but I continued prompting her.

'So tell me about the first time you did something to bring him to the attention of doctors,' I said.

'I can't remember much. He was asleep in his basket and I was in the kitchen. I was wrapping some ham in cling film. The thought just came to me, I can't believe I went through with it.'

She paused, as if thinking twice about finishing the story. I waited, not filling the gap.

'The cling film,' she croaked. 'I covered his face with it. And he went floppy.'

Emotions work four times faster than thought. Anger flared inside me, leaping unbidden from my stomach and swirling, tornado-like, up into my chest and throat. I swallowed hard and exhaled slowly, grappling to push the feeling back down. I remembered how useless I'd felt watching Callum's small pink body fitting; the image of the same child being smothered with cling film made me feel nauseous all over again.

As soon as Callum had stopped breathing, Adele had shouted to her mother to call 999 while she started to resuscitate him. She was referring to Callum as 'my son' again now, psychologically detaching herself from him as she had when talking to the paramedics at the mother-and-baby unit.

'I didn't do it for long. Not enough to seriously damage my son. I just...'

'Any length of time is too long,' I said steadily.

She looked taken aback but I never shy away from telling the truth to my clients. I'm not in the business of colluding with the distorted thinking that offenders adopt to excuse, minimize and, ultimately, give themselves permission to offend.

'And you did it for long enough to cause Callum to stop breathing, which could have caused irreversible brain damage,' I went on. My voice was soft but, as I spoke, I knew that my choice of words was coloured by my anger. 'Just as you contaminated his food enough to induce seizures and risk him going into cardiac arrest. It was luck, not judgement, that he didn't die.'

Medical maltreatment is considered one of the most lethal forms of child abuse, with 1 in 13 cases estimated to end in the child's death and a similar number of children left with permanent and life-limiting physical damage. I wanted to leave Adele with some food for thought but I was risking her shutting down.

She was quietly crying now. I asked her whether she had felt any satisfaction in assaulting Callum or had ever purposely inflicted pain or distress upon a child, or an animal, before.

'Of course not!' she cried, pushing an indignant tear from her cheek with the heel of her hand.

'I know that these are unpleasant questions but people harm children in this way for a variety of reasons and so it is important that I ask them,' I told her.

She nodded and we sat in an uneasy silence for a while.

'I just got hooked on it. That's what happened. But please believe me when I tell you I wasn't trying to hurt my boy. I felt disgusted with myself.'

'What was it that hooked you?'

She shot me a defeated look and shrugged as she said, 'Feeling important for once, I suppose.'

There it was. *Feeling important for once.* Adele had acted out a warped fusion of care and abuse of Callum in order to be viewed by others as both victim and hero, bravely caring for a worryingly sick child. In doing so, she'd won the notice and recognition she couldn't achieve in childhood.

She started crying again, burying her face in the crook of her arm.

'I used to fight with myself, I knew it wasn't right but I couldn't control it. I understand now that I have spoken to the psychiatrist that I've got Munchausen's by proxy and that it's an illness.'

You're not ill, you are self-serving, I thought. For a second, I thought I may even have said it out loud. The tornado was whirling around my chest again now and I breathed out another invisible, irritable cloud.

'I really want to get well, for Callum. My mum has found

a psychologist and I'm going to have therapy as soon as I get out. My mum is even seeing if she can pay for the psychologist to visit me here, if necessary. I'll do whatever it takes to get better, for Callum.'

I wondered if being told that she had a recognized kind of 'illness' was going to be more of a hindrance than a help to Adele. Generally speaking, I'm of the opinion that if someone finds it helpful to accept a psychiatric label as an explanation of their problems, that's fine. It's up to them how they choose to make sense of their experience. However, when the 'symptoms' of said 'illness' are abusing a child, it all becomes far too convenient.

'That's great. You are going to have a lot of work to do,' I told her.

Three weeks later, I was in my office, sifting through the week's referrals with Kathy, a wise and warm psychology assistant who was also part-way through her psychotherapy training. She had a wide smile and tight blonde curls that bounced as she spoke. My desk was littered with A4 envelopes and over-stuffed lever arch files wrapped in brown paper, criss-crossed with elastic bands. My cat, Bijou, had crammed himself into the nearest available space in a leather desk tray and was sound asleep.

The second package Kathy had opened was a request for an assessment of a mother in care proceedings – and the name was a familiar one. It was Justine and she was pregnant with her third child. With little support made available to her after Jasper's adoption, she hadn't yet made sufficient progress in her life to persuade social workers that she could care appropriately for her unborn child. She was already one of the 11,000 women – most of whom had become mothers when they were still children – who had had successive children removed from them between 2007 and 2014. I felt a stab of pessimism as I added the relevant assessment dates to my diary and locked Justine's paperwork into a filing cabinet. As we carried on sifting through the post, creating a tablecloth of manilla paper and mailing bags, the telephone rang, prompting Bijou to open his eyes just long enough to give me a dirty look.

It was the cut-glass tones of Adele's privately-funded solicitor. Ever courteous, he was calling to inform me of the outcome of her recent sentence hearing. Bucking the trend for increasingly harsh punishments for serious offences, the judge had handed Adele a two-year suspended sentence (a custodial sentence of sorts but with the jail time on hold with the condition she remained out of trouble and abided by the requirements that the judge chose to attach). She was ordered to attend the £100-an-hour psychological therapy arranged by her mother and not return to living at the family home. All future contact with Callum would be strictly managed by social services in collaboration with the psychologist and Adele's probation officer.

I thanked the solicitor for letting me know and hung up the phone. If I'd had a rubber chicken I would have given it a long, hard squeeze.

'She admitted to smothering a baby with cling film and apparently the judge commended her honesty!' I spat incredulously. 'A suspended sentence! UK law is clear that it is an act of medical abuse to fabricate or induce illness in a child, no matter what the reason. But she's got off lightly because the judge has been hoodwinked by a Munchausen syndrome by proxy diagnosis in mitigation.'

Kathy knew the details of Adele's case. 'But you didn't say she had that, did you?' she frowned.

'No, I didn't. But remember, I was specifically asked to address the opinion of the psychiatrist who did. I had to acknowledge that she *does* meet the diagnostic criteria – because she does – but I wrote a page-long addendum describing the problems with 'factitious disorder, etc.' as a diagnosis. It is a bullshit diagnosis and a sexist one at that!'

'How so?'

'It is 95 per cent women who get diagnosed with it. If it were a male pattern of behaviour, we would just call it what it is – abuse. But it is automatically assumed that a woman who does such a thing *must* be mentally disordered because it goes against all the expectations of our supposedly gentle, nurturing sex.'

Kathy asked me what I would have done if I were the judge. It was a good question. In considering my answer, I immediately began to simmer down and think more rationally.

'I have to admit,' I said. 'It *is* the best possible outcome for Callum. In fact, it is precisely the kind of creative sentencing that I advocate for and wish we had more of.'

'So why are you so angry? Or should I say, what emotion lies underneath the anger?' asked Kathy.

I raised an eyebrow. 'Are you giving me therapy, Kathy?'

'Only a little,' she winked.

'I'm frustrated,' I said. 'Adele is fragrant, feminine and oh-so-middle-class. Even her offences involved the use of Tupperware, and the cling film she used on Callum probably came in her mother's weekly Waitrose delivery! She can afford to pay privately for therapy. What chance would someone like Justine have had in her position?'

After Justine had been found with salt and laxatives, and within an hour of her shouting, 'You interfering bitch!' at the nurse, an on-call psychiatrist had been parachuted in and diagnosed her with borderline personality disorder (BPD) – a label that was first coined by psychiatrists who believed their patients to be 'bordering' on madness. Bordering. The diagnosis – as with all forms of personality disorder – is now widely synonymous with a special type of 'bad not mad'.

Justine may have preferred the equally applicable diagnosis of 'factitious disorder' but she didn't have the luxury of paying for the most helpfully obscuring label. And Justine wasn't well-mannered, softly spoken and contrite. She was 'difficult'. She swore. She could be gobby and might lob a loo roll at you.

The 'symptoms' of BPD include unstable relationships, shifting self-image, moodiness, impulsive, risky and self-harming behaviours, and feelings of emptiness and anger. It is a sticker loaded with negative connotations and in 2019, women and girls were seven times more likely to be saddled with it than men or boys displaying the same behaviours. An increasing number of psychologists argue that sexism explains the discrepancy. The loud expression of anger or distress is simply more socially acceptable in men, whose outbursts are more likely to be attributed to situational factors (i.e., having a bad day) than pathological character flaws. Robyn Timoclea, a researcher who also describes herself as a 'survivor' of a BPD diagnosis, found that clinicians often diagnose BPD in women based largely on judgements regarding their perceived social desirability.

Many of the women I've met while working for the Family Courts come with a 'borderline personality' stamp. It is hardly surprising. Most women fighting to cling onto their families would be likely, at some point, to hit enough of the diagnostic criteria to earn the badge. As might anyone traumatized by childhood neglect, abuse or exploitation, suffering domestic violence or dealing with any major stress or significant upheaval.

Justine might well meet the BPD criteria but at the same time she had rarely experienced consistent and caring acknowledgement of her needs, some of the means by which we learn to develop a positive sense of who we are and gain important emotional and social skills. Studies have shown that over 75 per cent of those diagnosed with BPD were subjected to abuse as children. So, if I had walked in her shoes, I would have likely bought that T-shirt too.

When writing Justine's report, I had been asked to set out recommendations for therapy that might enable her to safely care for Jasper. What she really needed was intense and proactive support to build a life that she didn't feel the need to escape from – a case of parenting the parent. That would require more than weekly therapy sessions. Even so, I set out a detailed plan of psychological work that could help her, though I knew that Justine would likely be on a waiting list for six months or longer, if she was offered anything at all. It was a timescale that was no use to her in terms of keeping Jasper, as the decision about his future would have to be made by then. Justine's BPD diagnosis might bump her up the list by a few weeks, but at what cost? It would also exclude her from many mental-health services that are allocated only to those who are 'ill' rather than personality 'disordered'. It is the stickiest of labels – official confirmation to both Justine and the court that she was fundamentally flawed and somehow different to others. Another chain around her neck that would follow her through any future proceedings she might face. And follow her it did. In years to come, I would see Justine again, when her fourth child was taken into care.

'Tea?' Kathy said, plonking the cat on my lap. I nodded gratefully, stroking Bijou as Kathy went to make me a cup of something strong but with lots of milk, exactly as I like it.

I thought about how, back in 1862, the French artist Gustave Doré had sketched a bust of the fictitious Baron Munchausen. It included a coat of arms bearing the motto 'Mendace Veritas' – In Lies, Truth.

When a mother feigns illness in herself or in her baby, there is always truth to be found among the lies. Sometimes you have to look very closely; other times it is staring you in the face.

The unpalatable truths about how our class, sex and social acceptability have the power to define and defend us are not so difficult to see.

CHAPTER FOUR
A FRANK CONFESSION

The news spread like wildfire. A man had been murdered on one of the largest and most impoverished housing estates on the outskirts of Rochdale.

It was late on Bonfire Night 2009 and most of the residents had gone home after enjoying a few fireworks and sparklers on the local recreation ground. They began spilling onto the streets again, and by the time the police arrived the estate was alive with gossip and commotion.

The victim was Ian Hayes, a car dealer in his fifties. Discovered half inside the doorway of his house, he had been battered about the head and both his kneecaps were shattered. It was 9.15pm and pitch dark by the time he was found. A small patch of overgrown garden separated Ian's house from the street and several people had walked past, mistaking the victim for a discarded 'penny for the guy' dummy.

Now an eerie, impromptu street party was breaking out as residents congregated outside their homes. Some of the teenagers launched rockets that lit up the black sky and neighbours huddled in packs, passing round cans of beer and slices of parkin. The bad-egg smell of burned sulphur percolated through the estate as tongues wagged and fingers started to point.

Ian was well known to the police for attempts to sell 'cut and shut' cars with fake documents.

'The police will have their work cut out finding who did it,' neighbours tutted. 'Anyone who's ever done business with that fella has a motive...'

The grapevine rapidly grew the speculation into fake news: the victim had had it coming for years, they said. It was no surprise that, finally, a customer he'd ripped off had killed him out of revenge.

Except it wasn't one of Ian's unhappy customers who slid swiftly into the frame. Milling through the crowds that night was 21-year-old Frank Eccleston, a quiet young man who lived two streets away from the scene of the crime with his dad, stepmum and eight-year-old half-sister, Holly. Frank was widely regarded in the community as being 'a bit strange'. The fact that he had less fat on him than a stick of celery but liked to dress like an aspiring Hell's Angel – think a faux-leather version of Meat Loaf's character Eddie in *The Rocky Horror Picture Show* – did nothing to enhance his reputation.

Frank's behaviour that night was odder than usual, it seemed. With residents on red alert and all the nearby Sherlocks and Miss Marples on the lookout for clues, this didn't go unnoticed.

'He's been darting about, looking agitated,' one person reported to the police.

'He's been acting even more weirdly than usual,' another said.

Once the local drums had started up, the banging became deafening. Neighbours were lining up to give their two penn'orth about Frank's suspicious behaviour.

Of course, these flimsy observations were no grounds for arrest, but then Frank himself decided to make life easy for the investigating officers. Sidling up to a group of boys who were attempting to light a Catherine wheel, he made an unexpected confession. 'I done it,' he said. 'I killed him.'

The first I knew of the case was when Frank's solicitor collared me as I came out of a meeting with another client at her firm. I'd worked with her for five years, almost as long as I'd been self-employed, and she'd always reminded me of a terrier, with her delicate, pointed features and high-pitched, yappy voice. I'd definitely want her on my team if I were in trouble because she sprang into action immediately and was tenacious once she'd caught the scent of a defence strategy. Almost before I knew what was happening, she'd steered me inside her office and was handing me a brown envelope. Frank had been interviewed twice by police, she explained, and she had serious concerns about how both sessions had been conducted.

The first interview had taken place in the early hours of 6 November. Frank was standing by his confession and had declined his right to legal representation. The second interview came four days later, this time with both a duty solicitor and an 'appropriate adult' present – a designated person assigned to support him and make sure he fully understood what was happening.

'I need a quick turnaround assessment of both interviews,' the solicitor barked at me. 'And an expert opinion regarding my client's vulnerability.' Doubting that I would be allowed to leave the building without accepting the challenge, I picked up the bone.

The following day, I cleared as much as I could from my diary and peeled open the envelope that she had given me. Inside were a slim wad of papers and two CDs of the video recordings of the interviews, made so recently there were no transcripts available yet. I loaded up the first interview. The quality of the footage was typically grainy. The camera pointed in the direction of the interviewee, capturing the backs, shoulders and bald spots of the two interviewing police officers.

Frank's *Rocky Horror Picture Show* outfit had been taken from him as evidence and he was wearing joggers and a plastic-looking sweatshirt that swamped his stick-thin body. Even dressed head to toe in concrete grey he still managed to stand out, sporting as he did a dated mullet and the strangest goatee I'd ever seen. It had length but no substance, like stretched candyfloss.

Frank's eyes were darting round his head and he was taking sharp gulps of breath.

'Yeah, I did it,' he said. 'I did Mr Hayes.'

'Where did this all take place?'

'In his front garden, that's where I did it.'

'Talk us through what happened there, Frank.'

'Well, I battered him, that's all.'

'You say you battered him?'

'Yes. I killed him. Battered him.'

'How did you batter him?'

'Erm...with my bare hands it was, honest.'

The police officer closest to the camera turned his head to glance at his colleague. The minimal information Frank gave didn't tally with what little detail they already had at this point, because a trail of blood had shown that the attack had started in Ian's kitchen and it was clear from his injuries that some sort of weapon had been used.

'Can you explain more about what happened? What time do you think it was when you arrived at Mr Hayes's house?'

Frank started crying, pulling his elbows tight to his torso and flapping his hands, the way you do in front of your mouth when you've eaten something too hot.

'Alright, son, is there anything you want to tell us about why you would do something like this?'

At this question, Frank's voice became louder and higher. 'So you will tell my dad,' he said. 'So you will tell my dad.'

It wasn't clear if Frank was asking a question or stating a fact.

'Tell your dad?' the interviewer repeated.

Frank looked directly at him. 'I'm a serial killer,' he declared.

The officers didn't know how to take this. 'What do you mean by "I'm a serial killer"?'

'I don't know,' he mumbled, wiping his nose with the sleeve of his sweatshirt. 'I don't know what I said it for.' He didn't seem to grasp the potential ramifications of claiming to be a multiple murderer while under police caution.

It must have been rapidly dawning on the police that Frank might be classed as 'vulnerable' in this situation and, as such, there was somebody important missing from the room. It is the custody sergeant's responsibility to identify anybody with even a hint of 'mental vulnerability' (the bar for which is set deliberately low to reflect the fact that police personnel are not, and cannot be expected to be, mental-health experts) and ensure that they are interviewed in the company of an appropriate adult. An interview taking place without this critical safeguard breaches the Police and Criminal Evidence Act 1984 (PACE) Codes of Practice, risking any evidence gained being rendered inadmissible in court, not to mention the possibility of disciplinary action.

I could just picture the colourful thought bubbles above the interviewing officers' heads, cursing their custody sergeant. I wouldn't want to be in any of their shoes when the Terrier got hold of them.

Still, the police pressed on, asking Frank to take them through the earlier events of the night. He explained there had been a small Bonfire Night party at his house with his immediate family and some of his cousins. 'But then I had an argument with someone and ran off.'

As soon as he said this, Frank jumped out of his seat. His head and shoulders were no longer in frame on the video but it was clear from the way his body was jolting, and the way the officers leaped up and around the table that separated them, that he was banging his head against the wall. The interview was brought to an abrupt close, having lasted just 36 minutes.

Frank was bailed without charge but, now with unmissable clues to his distressed state, transferred directly to a 'place of safety', namely the local acute psychiatric ward.

Three days later, the 'murder victim' was sitting up in his hospital bed. Ian Hayes needed two total knee replacements and he had a very nasty headache but he definitely wasn't dead. He may have looked as lifeless as a stuffed guy when he was found but it turned out he was still breathing when the ambulance arrived – a detail lost in the rumours billowing like black smoke around the estate.

Not only had Ian survived, he was already well enough to tell the police that the son of one of his neighbours – Frank Eccleston – had broken into the back of his house and, when confronted, had attacked him in the kitchen with a baseball bat. Ian couldn't offer any explanation as to why Frank would do this but he did tell police that everyone on the estate knew he was 'probably just an accident waiting to happen' because he was 'strange' and 'always talking about serial killers'.

Ian's statement was a breakthrough moment. Until then, the police didn't have a shred of physical evidence tying Frank to the attack; nothing had been found on his clothes to link him to either the victim or the crime scene. However, a neighbour three streets away had found a bloodstained baseball bat stuffed in her garden hedge, which had been sent off for forensic testing.

With Frank's initial account having more holes in it than a mint Aero, the police were keen to get him back in for questioning. But, not wanting to repeat their first mistake, this time he was accompanied by his father, Frank Snr, acting as appropriate adult.

When I pressed play on the second interview video, I had to pull the computer screen closer to my face just to confirm what I was seeing. Frank Jnr appeared to be wearing the most inappropriate T-shirt you could imagine. There, grinning from his chest, was a mug shot of the American serial killer John Wayne Gacy. I was momentarily distracted, wondering why any company would want to manufacture such a thing (I've since discovered there is a thriving market for serial-killer couture, and indeed every type of distasteful memorabilia, with websites dedicated to the sale of crime-scene pictures, personal effects, handwritten letters and so on).

Returning my focus to the screen in front of me, I realized Frank's T-shirt wasn't the only thing that stood out as incongruous. The police interviewer was only part way through the caution when Frank Snr began to make his presence known.

'But if you go to court and say something there which you have not told me about, and they think you could have told me, it may harm your case. Anything you do say may be…'

'Don't tell them what you did, son,' Frank Snr ordered, jabbing the elbow of his heavily tattooed left arm – the only part of his body visible on screen – into Frank Jnr's ribs.

I couldn't help but laugh. It reminded me of that ageless *Dad's Army* scene where the German captain barks at Pike,

'Your name will also go on the list! What is it?' only for Captain Mainwaring to wade in with the brilliant piece of advice: 'Don't tell him, Pike.'

Almost anybody over the age of 18 can act as an appropriate adult, although they are most often parents or guardians, social workers or specifically trained volunteers. They are only meant to intervene in the interview if they feel that the person they are supporting is being unfairly treated or needs help to fully participate. The type of 'advice' that Frank Snr was dispensing is most certainly not in the role description.

As the interview progressed, the police were not covering themselves in glory either. Since Ian had been so confident in identifying Frank as his attacker, they were more inclined to accept Frank's confession than they had been the first time round. So inclined, in fact, they were practically leading Frank into Ian's kitchen and putting the weapon in his hand.

'What did you hit Ian Hayes with?'

'Nothing...I mean hands, my fists.'

'That's not true, is it?'

'I don't know.'

'Look at him!' Frank Snr interjected. 'He is only seven stone when wet, of course it's not true.'

'Please, Mr Eccleston, let him speak. Frank, I think you are getting upset now because you know you did something more serious than hit him with your fists, didn't you?'

'I suppose so.'

'Did you hit him with something like a stick? Or a baseball bat?'

'A stick...baseball bat,' Frank said, just loud enough to be heard over his dad's irritated huffing.

'So you are saying now that you hit him with a baseball bat, is that right?'

'Yeah, I went round to his house and battered him with a baseball bat, didn't I?'

In what I suspect were genuine efforts to 'help' their floundering suspect tell them what they already believed to be true, the officers were making a whole new set of blunders. There were moments when they strayed into blatantly coercive interrogation tactics by asking leading questions, suggesting a 'correct' answer and repeating the questioning until Frank eventually complied. I could only imagine the mixture of both horror and glee that the Terrier must have felt when she first saw these recordings. They were a case study in how *not* to interview a vulnerable suspect and she would have a strong argument to have them dismissed as evidence. The police had displayed exactly the kind of bad practice that PEACE, the UK's conversational and non-confrontational police interviewing model, is designed to eliminate.[1] PEACE was introduced in the nineties after a series of unsound convictions were overturned. You stray from that interview

---

[1] The letters stand for preparation/planning; explaining the purpose of the interview; asking for the suspect's account of the evidence/what happened; challenging their account/concluding; evaluation. Every operational officer in the country gets PEACE training and officers use this framework to ensure that as much useful information as possible is gathered in the interview process.

framework at your peril. My analysis was going to make embarrassing reading for the police.

After his second interview, Frank had been bailed again and returned to the hospital. He was due to return to the police station in two weeks' time, when officers hoped to be able to charge him. However, if the Terrier got her way *and* if Frank would accept her advice to keep schtum when she accompanied him in his third interview, the police and CPS might only have the victim's account to work with. And that is not as cut and dried as you might expect, given that when a person is suddenly confronted by an assailant and knocked unconscious, it is easy to argue for a case of mistaken identity.

The hospital Frank was in had a newly refurbished psychiatric unit with male and female wards on either side of a large square communal area that was painted pastel green and lined with flame-retardant shiny purple chairs in various shapes and sizes.

Before I'd even been let in, I spotted Frank through the glass in the door, hovering next to the nurses' office. You couldn't miss him. He was wearing the same John Wayne Gacy T-shirt he had on in the police interview, a black leather-like biker jacket, jeans ripped at the knees and one fingerless leather glove. Through the rips in the jeans, you could see his bony knees and pipe-cleaner legs.

'Are you the psychologist?' he said as soon as he saw me.

'I am, yes.'

'You are Kerry Daynes, consultant forensic psychologist. I am Frank Eccleston, studying BTEC HNC computing at college and detained under section 2 of the Mental Health Act 1983.'

'Well, hello, Frank.'

'That means that I am being assessed and can stay here for up to 28 days,' he added, helpfully.

I'd normally want to have a good sift through a person's hospital notes before I saw them, but I could see Frank was champing at the bit to get started. I popped into the nurses' office to quickly ask if there was anything I needed to know. It was his first admission I was told and, no, there wasn't much to tell. Frank had been quiet since he arrived, he'd refused to see his family when they dropped off some clothes for him and he had spent that night in his room pacing and flapping his hands. Other than that, he seemed 'settled' and keen to follow the ward routine. 'That's about it,' the nurse said. As I thanked her and turned to leave, she suddenly remembered something else. 'Oh, just one other thing – he's been asked to stop telling other patients facts about serial killers.'

A nursing assistant walked me and Frank to a visitors' room, a place we could have some privacy. We passed through the communal area where a group of patients were passing the time. A girl in a grey jumper with a big red heart on it was sitting at a table, playing Jenga with an older woman. Next to her was a man snoring softly in a chair and another man was standing up close by, listening intently to a CD on a portable player. 'Task two,' I heard a disembodied voice say in a strong Spanish accent. 'How do I get to the bus station? *¿Cómo llego a la estación de autobuses?*' The man held a clutch of CDs in his hand. He was obviously hoping to get a lot further than the bus station, I thought.

I'd planned some basic psychometric tests, which are essential to this sort of assessment. I thought I'd start with them, giving myself and Frank some time to get comfortable with each other before the quizzing became more personal. I explained to him that I was carrying out the Wechsler Adult Intelligence Scale – Fourth Edition (WAIS-IV), the most globally accepted measure of IQ (intelligence quotient).

This hefty bit of kit comes in a briefcase – not dissimilar in weight to the Wechsler Memory Scales assessment I used with Clifford – but there are more props to juggle with this one, such as jigsaws, thick puzzle books and building blocks used to test a person's abstract problem-solving and visual–motor skills. The assessment has 15 parts to it, all designed to tap into different domains of intelligence. Frank stopped gazing around the room and began to concentrate intently. He got off to a shaky start with a vocabulary test but when I asked him to arrange the set of red and white blocks to match a pattern shown on a card, he whizzed through the set. 'What's next?' he asked enthusiastically, still staring at the cubes in front of him.

The arithmetic subtest was a particular favourite of his.

'George gives eight people four cards each. He has six cards left for tomorrow. How many cards did he have all together?'

You have 30 seconds to complete each question but Frank answered almost immediately.

'Thirty-eight.'

'Good job, Frank.'

'Moses Sithole killed 30 people. Ian Brady was born on 2 January 1938.'

I hadn't expected to be regaled with this extra information, but I didn't pass comment.

'If eight machines can finish a job in six days, how many machines are needed to finish a job in half a day?'

This time Frank thought for 23 seconds before giving the correct answer: 'Ninety-six.'

I was quite envious at his maths skills, to be honest, having needed three attempts to pass GCSE maths and make it to university.

'William Bonin was executed on 23 February 1996.'

Clearly, Frank was also much better versed in serial-killer trivia than I was. He had a fact for nearly every question, all 22 of them.

'That's some pretty impressive knowledge you have there,' I said when the arithmetic subtest was done. 'What do you like about serial killers?'

'I just like them.'

I asked him what he liked about the man who was leering at me from his T-shirt.

'John Wayne Gacy was born on 17 March 1942, he killed 33 people, he was sentenced to death on 13 March 1980 and was executed by lethal injection on 10 May 1994. His last words were "Kiss my ass".'

Interestingly, Frank didn't tell me any of the usual headline-grabbing details surrounding Gacy, such as the fact he tortured, raped and strangled his victims, mostly runaway boys, or became known as the 'Killer Clown'. Nor did he want to engage me in conjecture about Gacy's motive, typically an irresistible focal point of any discussion about serial killers, and therefore the reason I am invited to dinner parties. (Serial killers tend to have multiple motives, incidentally, which may change over time and may not be fully understood even by themselves.)

Though it's not an ideal hobby to advertise when you find yourself under suspicion for attempted murder, Frank's obvious fascination with serial killers wasn't so unusual. Serial killers have captivated the general public ever since so-called 'Jack the Ripper' terrorized the streets of Whitechapel in 1888. Though more than 130 years have passed since the killings of Polly Nichols, Annie Chapman, Elizabeth Stride, Mary Jane Kelly and Catherine Eddowes, their unidentified killer has become the stuff of myth and legend, the top hat and cloak-wearing figure the subject of a continuing stream of books, films, documentaries and London sightseeing tours. On Halloween at the Jack the Ripper Museum, you can even take a cheeky selfie with a model of one of the victim's corpses, as though this was nothing more than a Gothic horror fairytale to shiver at, rather than a glorification of the real-life destruction of women.

Whether serial killers are long dead or very much alive and locked up in the prison down the road, it seems that we can't be shown too much or invited to speculate too far about this particular brand of criminal. If you look at the number of true-crime documentaries on the subject, you'd think they were more common than house burglars but I can currently count on my fingers and a few toes the number of serial killers in prison in England and Wales.

Scott Bonn, professor of criminology at Drew University, New Jersey, and the author of *Why We Love Serial Killers,* explains why this tiny percentage of the criminal population attracts so much attention. 'Serial killers tantalize, terrify and entertain the public,' he writes. 'Since at least the 1970s they have been frequent and chilling actors on centre stage in the news and entertainment media. Massive and highly stylized news coverage of real life serial killers such as David Berkowitz, Ted Bundy, and Jeffrey Dahmer transforms them into ghoulish popular culture celebrities.'

It strikes me that the victims of serial killers don't share in this elevated status. The public's appetite for their lives, beyond gory and titillating details of the violence they were subjected to, is negligible. We often don't recall their names and even if we do, they are relegated to bit parts in the serial-killer stage show.

At 12.29pm, Frank became anxious that he would be late for lunch, which was due to be served at 12.30. I took him back to the communal space and, while I was there, helped myself to a cup of cold tea dispensed from a machine in the corner. The game of Jenga had ended but the girl in the heart jumper was still there, sitting quietly next to the Spanish student and an older man who was giving an inaudible running commentary of something he was reading in the *Racing Post.*

I left Frank waiting for his lunch and totted up the results of his assessment as I ate a cheese and onion sandwich I'd picked up from the hospital Costa on my way in. Frank had an overall IQ score of 86, which falls in the low-average range (the average score being 100). He didn't have a learning disability but his full-scale IQ was not the best way to describe his abilities, as his subtest scores were distinctly uneven.

When most people's WAIS-IV subtest scores are plotted onto a graph, they appear as a wavy line. But Frank's scores were so up and down that they reminded me of the Manhattan skyline. His best performance had, unsurprisingly, been on the measure of his mathematical abilities. Sitting far below that was his score on the comprehension subtest, a measure of his understanding of social rules, conventions and expressions. I was beginning to understand the nature of Frank's 'vulnerability'.

After lunch, we moved on to the Gudjonsson Suggestibility Scales (GSS), another well-used psychometric test. This one does what it says on the tin, measuring two different aspects of 'interrogative suggestibility'. The first is how much a person being questioned *yields* to leading questions; the second measures how much the subject *shifts* their responses when some mild interrogative thumbscrews are applied.

I read out a short story to Frank as he picked at one of the rips in his jeans. Then I asked him to tell me what he could remember without any prompting, which was most of it, despite him looking wholeheartedly uninterested.

'How many questions are there?' he asked.

'Twenty.'

'Harold Shipman hanged himself at 6.20am on 13 January 2004.'

'Yes, he did,' I acknowledged, before moving swiftly on.

We worked our way through the questions about the story, 15 of which were 'suggestive' and five 'neutral'. The GSS confirmed what I'd seen in his second police interview, with Frank falling hard for leading questions. Not only that, his 'shift' score for changing his answers when he was told he'd made a mistake was significantly above average.

I now had all the numbers required to prove that Frank was a particularly likely candidate to offer unreliable information when subjected to bad-practice police interviewing. He didn't know it, but his incriminating statements were looking increasingly unlikely to ever make it in front of a jury.

All of this also meant that I needed to be especially careful to document everything I asked him throughout the remainder of my assessment and not to lead him in any way. And with that in mind, I decided it was time to call it a day, so that I could go home and plan the rest of my questions.

'I don't know about you but my head is spinning with all that we've got through today,' I said.

'No, it isn't,' Frank replied bluntly.

'What I meant is, all these facts and information have given me a bit of a headache. You've done brilliantly but let's stop now and we can meet again tomorrow.'

I put my coat on, packed up my briefcase and Frank and I walked out of the visitors' room and through the communal area together, on the way back to the nurses' office.

That's when a fine spray of something warm and wet hit the side of my face, completely out of nowhere.

As I turned my head, a jet of sticky liquid with a sharp metallic taste shot straight into my mouth, coating my bottom lip.

The girl in the grey jumper was standing beside me, holding both her hands above her head, as if surrendering to police. Her lips were moving but no sound was coming out and her eyebrows were pulled together in an expression of terror. In her right hand was a shard of broken CD and the wrist of her other arm was as ruby red as the heart on her jumper. Lively shots of blood were firing from a deep cut, straight across the radial artery. I'd seen plenty of self-inflicted wounds in the past but few as life-threatening as this.

It's surprising how fast your reactions kick in when you see fresh blood escaping a person's body. I did a lot of things, seemingly all at once. I dropped my briefcase, snatched the broken piece of CD out of the girl's hand, shoved it in my coat pocket and reached for her cut wrist.

'I'm just going to take hold of your wrist,' I said, though I'd already grabbed it with both hands before I finished my sentence. I started squeezing as tight as I could, applying pressure to stem the flow of blood.

I didn't have an emergency alarm on me, but then again I didn't have a hand free anyway to activate it. 'Hellopo!' I bellowed, my adrenaline-fuelled amalgamation of 'help' and 'hello'.

'I didn't mean to,' the girl gasped, tears streaming down her face.

As gently as I could, I told her, 'I know. It's OK. Did you just want the horrible feeling to stop?'

She nodded.

'Now, put your other hand with mine and press as hard as you can.' This time my voice came out sounding more matronly. I didn't want to alarm her but I needed as much help as I could to apply pressure to the wound.

She did as I asked. 'That's it,' I said. 'Well done.'

By now, a male member of staff had run out of one of the offices behind us, silently sidling up beside the girl and gripping hold of her elbow.

'Get off me,' she shrieked, jerking violently in the opposite direction, pulling me with her as she tried to push him away.

I was filled with an urge to scream, 'Get off her' too but I wasn't on my own territory and, whoever he was, the man wasn't part of my team to instruct. All I could do was hang on to the girl's wrist as best I could, my knuckles going white with the effort.

I wasn't letting go, but evidently nor was he. We were both pulled forwards, backwards and sideways as the girl continued trying to shake him off. It was while the three of us performed this bizarre Hokey Cokey that I felt another unwelcome sensation. This time it was that unstoppable falling feeling, the one that makes your heart leap and your mouth go dry because you know you've already gone beyond the tipping point and there is no way of stopping the inevitable.

As I fell to the floor my hand was wrenched from the girl's wrist. We all landed in a tangled heap, blood spurting onto the shiny lino as the girl crashed on her bottom and I fell half on top of the man, who was round and hairy and smelled of Deep Heat and cigarettes.

A couple of nurses had appeared. Both were wearing blue disposable plastic gloves and one was opening a First Aid kit. As I rolled out of my unseemly position to let them get to work I could hear the nurses talking softly to the girl, who was sobbing. I was on my hands and knees now, breathlessly disentangling my visitor's badge from the lower buttons of the man's shirt.

'How was it for you?' he grinned.

I gave an involuntary half smile and took his hand as he pulled me up off the floor. I handed him the slice of CD in my pocket.

'Celine Dion?' the man whispered conspiratorially. 'Makes me want to slit my wrist too.'

I gave him the other half of my smile.

Suddenly remembering I'd been with Frank, I turned to see where he was. To my surprise, he'd slid down the wall a couple of metres away and was sitting with his knobbly knees pointing up to the ceiling and his eyes closed. His hands were in front of his face, flapping wildly, and he'd taken on a deathlike pallor.

I knelt down next to him. 'Frank, are you OK?'

He squeezed his shoulders in, to make himself smaller. 'Don't touch me with it,' he said in a high voice. 'I hate blood. Don't get it on me.'

'Don't worry, there's none on you. Everybody is going to be alright. Let's get you up and get you back to your ward.'

I backed off as the hairy man dropped to his haunches, lifted Frank's arm around his shoulder and helped him to his feet. I watched as Frank was half carried away, looking like a limp lettuce leaf falling out the side of a Big Mac.

'Why did she do that?' I heard him say. 'I feel sick.'

Meanwhile, I was thinking how curious it was that my allegedly aspiring serial killer – in the frame for a violent and undoubtedly messy assault – was afraid of blood.

To their credit, the hospital had a decent 'critical incident debrief' system. Before I'd had the chance to sit down with another cup of cold tea, one of their therapy team, a cognitive-behavioural nurse specialist, came to check that I was alright. I always find it a bit awkward to be on the receiving end of any kind of debrief but I don't think the nurse noticed my unease. She was very focused on working her way down a form of questions about how I was feeling about what just happened (I didn't know, I hadn't had time to work it out yet) and whether I needed any further support (I didn't, I had that covered by my regular supervision meetings).

The last question was, 'Is there anything more I can do to help you today?'

'Actually, yes there is,' I found myself saying. 'Frank, who I am here to see and is detained for assessment…well, it's beyond the scope of my job, but do you have anyone here who is specifically trained in the assessment of adults who may be on the autistic spectrum?'

The nurse told me there was someone trained in carrying out specialist assessments at the hospital and she would see what she could do.

Autistic spectrum 'disorder' (ASD, or autistic spectrum *difference* as I like to think of it) is a wide-ranging category of brain-based variations that show themselves mostly in a person's ability to correctly 'read' others, creating difficulties in communication and navigating the social world. The number of people diagnosed with ASD has soared over the last 30 years, due in no small part to our awareness of it being piqued by the furore surrounding the MMR vaccine and the success of films like *Rain Man*.

The World Health Organization estimates that worldwide, 0.6 per cent of people are on the autistic spectrum, with 1 in 160 children potentially being diagnosed with ASD. In the UK at least, it seems too many of them end up in secure psychiatric hospitals, where its prevalence is estimated at 2.3 per cent. Yet autism can often go undetected, slipping through the gap between learning disabilities and mental-health diagnoses (or being misattributed to either). If someone is referred for assessment in the UK, NICE Quality Standards set a target of no more than three months' waiting time for the first appointment. However, in reality, the average waiting time for an adult is two years.

Hopefully Frank wouldn't have to wait that long. I wouldn't normally rush to have somebody like him, who appeared to be on the milder side of the autistic spectrum, diagnosed (after all, *vive la différence!*). But not knowing where his current legal problems might end, it seemed wise to seize an opportunity.

If my head was spinning at the end of Frank's psychometric testing, it was whirling like a dervish by the time I got home that night. I took off my bloodstained coat and put it straight in the bin, wondering how the girl was doing now. I thought back over Frank's reaction to her slit wrist, as well as his *Mastermind*-worthy knowledge of the minutiae of serial killers' lives. Special interests are one of the most common characteristics of people with autism, but I wanted to understand what serial killers represented to Frank. It was a thought that bubbled in my brain all night.

In 1990, Sture Bergwall confessed to the abduction, rape and murder of 11-year-old Johan Asplund, a boy whose mysterious disappearance more than a decade earlier had led to Sweden's biggest missing-child case of its time. Bergwall was a patient at Säter secure psychiatric hospital, and quickly began to confess to many more murders – 39, all told. Having changed his name to Thomas Quick (his supposed sinister alter ego), he admitted to not only dispatching his victims but eating their remains.

The newspapers inevitably named him 'the cannibal' and declared that Sweden had spawned its own real-life Hannibal Lecter. Thomas Quick did not object. On the contrary, he revelled in the media spotlight, or at least he did for a time. Curiously, after being convicted of eight of the murders, Quick suddenly stopped cooperating with the police. Not only that, he reverted to his original name and all but disappeared inside the walls of Säter.

The unusual turn of events roused the interest of an award-winning investigative journalist, Hannes Råstam. After picking over 50,000 pages of court documents, police interviews and therapy notes, Råstam was astonished by what he found – or rather by what he didn't find. There was not one shred of physical or technical evidence for any of Bergwall's convictions. No DNA, no murder weapons linking to him, no eyewitness accounts that stood up. Unbelievably, Sweden's apparently most prolific serial killer had been convicted on the strength of his confessions alone. When Råstam confronted Bergwall with his findings, he then made the most astonishing confession of all: he had made the whole thing up.

The 'why' is what interested me. It's one of the questions Bergwall was asked in an interview he gave to *The Observer* in 2012, towards the end of his incarceration at Säter.

Bergwall was originally sent to the hospital after participating in an armed robbery. He was 'a very lonely person' when the lies started, he said. 'It was about belonging to something. I was in a place with violent criminals and I noticed that the worse or more violent or serious the crime, the more interest someone got from the psychiatric personnel. I also wanted to belong to that group, to be an interesting person in here.'

Bergwall more than succeeded, achieving such a degree of celebrity status within the hospital that he was described by one staff member as 'almost a Jesus figure'. Along with his notoriety came unlimited access to therapy and benzodiazepine, a mind-altering tranquillizer. His team of therapists used an intense, experimental (not to mention highly dubious and since discredited) psychotherapy that claimed to reveal repressed memories. Bergwall delivered in spades, inventing a horrific history of child abuse. Then, taking inspiration from *American Psycho*, *Silence of the Lambs* and newspaper reports of unsolved murders, he concocted false confession after false confession.

In the 2015 documentary film *The Confessions of Thomas Quick,* he admitted that the more grotesque the details he shared, the more pleased the therapist was, and so the more he invented. It was only when a new doctor arrived and took him off the heavy drugs he'd been on for years that Bergwall stopped telling lies and began to finally face the truth.

In hindsight, it had been a perfect storm. A lost and lonely man, desperate to belong and be noticed at any cost. Ambitious, misguided therapists courting the kudos of an intense study into the sadistic serial-killer mind. Investigating police officers hungry for the glory of cracking a serial-killer case.

Bergwall was released in 2013, having been acquitted of all eight murder convictions.

It's not just psychiatric patients who want to align themselves with notorious killers for personal or professional gain. There's a whole raft of self-styled experts and talking-head 'psychologists' who have never actually spoken to a serial killer but pop up regularly in TV documentaries or at a theatre near you. Tapping into the Hollywood stereotype, they promise to take you 'inside the mind' of a serial killer and answer such fallacious questions as 'What drives someone to end another person's life as easily as cutting grass?' (Believe it or not, serial killers frequently feel intense conflict about their activities.)

One example is Paul Harrison, a former police officer from Kettering who called himself the world's number-one serial-killer expert. He claimed to have access to a long list of high-profile killers and, knowing that I've met a number in the course of my work, once emailed me to ask if I was interested in working on some joint projects with him.

Naturally, I asked Harrison how he'd managed to spend time with so many of the world's most talked-about offenders, including Ted Bundy, Levi Bellfield, Jeffrey Dahmer and (funnily enough) John Wayne Gacy.

'It wasn't easy,' he said.

It can't have been – some of the people Harrison claimed to have interviewed in his 33 books were already dead at the time he was supposed to have met them.

He toured the country with a sell-out show, promoted with the slogan, 'I tell them "I'm not your friend, I'm your conscience"'. I discovered that he was also telling audience members that we were good friends. It was all news to me. I'd never even met the man.

Harrison's downfall came in 2019 after he claimed Peter Sutcliffe had told him, 'You seem completely indifferent to me. I'm scared of you.' When Sutcliffe got wind of this, he said he had never met Harrison, calling him a charlatan and a con man. 'What a wazzock he is,' were apparently his exact words, which sound far more authentic than Harrison's supposed quote. The cop-turned-showman fell on his sword, cancelling his events and apologizing for letting people down. Even if you didn't set yourself up as a serial-killer expert, it's hard to imagine a worse humiliation than having your reputation trashed by Peter Sutcliffe…

The morning after the Hokey Cokey debacle, I woke up with a bruised hip and painful knee from where I'd landed on the floor. What little sleep I'd had was disturbed by images of blood and I'd woken with a start as I dreamed I was falling. It was dark and I would have liked to make an executive decision to stay tucked underneath my duvet, but I was going back to the hospital to finish off my work with Frank.

I hobbled downstairs, put the kettle on and opened my tea cupboard as usual. I don't always pay attention to the nine-inch-high plastic figure who stands alongside my catering-sized pack of Yorkshire teabags (when you drink as much tea as I do, there's no point faffing around with small boxes). But today I took a good, long look at her.

The poised and confident figure represents my 'inner warrior'. She's some sort of anime cartoon character, bought for me by a friend who said it reminded her of me. That must be because of the long red hair and comedy breasts because, alas, I don't own a floor-length black battle gown or a red-handled samurai sword. Still, I identify with this figure and have adopted her as my imagined inner helper. When the need arises, she reminds me to dust myself down, pick myself up and power through. She also encourages me to work for what I believe in and what I want to achieve, and to rest when I should.

I sometimes use imagery in therapy sessions, encouraging clients to create their own inner helper. It doesn't matter if it's a physical figure that stands next to their teabags or a vision that exists solely inside their head. The important thing is it represents strength, wisdom, kindness, nurturing or whatever that individual needs to keep them on track. Crucially, an inner helper doesn't have human frailties, so it can never let you down or fail to say what you need to hear when you are distressed. I've known people to conjure all kinds of imaginary helpers. Mother Earth-type figures are popular, as are strong, historical characters like Joan of Arc. Tigers and other powerful animals are common, too, though one patient surprised me by choosing Basil Brush. Whatever floats your boat!

I identify with my inner helper because warriors have defeats as well as victories and they remind us it's acceptable to be wounded. Clients who've been subjected to abuse often tell me they don't want to be called a 'victim', though neither do they feel like a 'survivor'. Warrior is a much better fit, they say, and I understand that.

That morning, my inner warrior reminded me that it was Friday and that I just needed to get through today, complete Frank's assessment and then have the weekend off. Instead of dwelling on my aching bones and lost sleep I refocused on the task in hand.

I wanted to get a glimpse into how Frank viewed himself and how he saw the world and so today, in addition to my usual questions, I was going to use a Repertory Grid Technique. Based on George Kelly's 'personal construct' theory, it's a method of teasing out information about how a person looks at life. Most importantly, it allows the person to use entirely their own language to articulate the meaning they attach to people, objects and events. There would be no chance of my putting words into Frank's mouth.

I was pleased to find that he seemed to have made a full recovery from the shock of the previous day and grateful that he had gone for an all-black, studded ensemble this morning so I didn't have to spend any more time eyeball to eyeball with John Wayne Gacy.

After lunch, I started with a quick demonstration of how repertory grids work and then we moved on to the topic of 'Frank, and the important people in his life'.

Between us, we chose a set of 'elements': Frank (as I am now), Frank (as I'd like to be), Frank Snr (his dad), Jenny (his stepmum), Holly (his half-sister) plus some other people whom Frank listed as important, including, of course, serial killers. Frank sat bolt upright in his chair, in anticipation of this becoming a far more interesting part of the assessment than anything that had gone before it.

Then we worked our way methodically through the most important part of the technique. Using different combinations of the people who made up our list of elements, Frank was asked to compare and contrast them to each other until eventually he had generated a list of ideas describing how he experienced them. Frank's list, known as 'constructs', included:

Strong – Weak
Scary – Nice
Clever – Stupid
Shouts a lot – Is quiet
In charge – Has to do as they are told
People pay attention to them – People laugh at them.

To finish, Frank was asked to rate each person against each construct, on a scale of one to five.

What emerged was that he rated serial killers as the most 'strong', 'scary' and 'clever' of all people. They were 'in charge', Frank believed, and 'people pay attention to them'. This confirmed what was already obvious – that Frank was mightily impressed by serial killers, or, should I say, he was enamoured with their media-spun image. In reality, serial killers are not evil geniuses. Those who have had their IQs tested fall between borderline and just above average intelligence – the same as the general population. And while it's true that many serial killers seek power, control and domination over victims, more often than not this is to compensate for profound inadequacies. Until their crimes catch up with them, nearly all are viewed by those around them as innocuous, unassuming and therefore of little interest. I was tempted to tell Frank all this but it wasn't the time, and would have felt like informing a five-year-old that Father Christmas doesn't exist.

In sharp contrast, Frank saw himself at the other end of the scale to serial killers, rating himself as the most 'weak' person of all. He was someone who 'had to do as they are told', the person 'people laugh at' and 'don't pay any attention to'. Like his half-sister, Holly, he said he was 'quiet' and 'frightened'. But unlike Holly, Frank as he would *like* to be was 'strong', 'scary' and 'in charge' – attributes he also rated Frank Snr highly on, along with 'shouts a lot'.

But that is not all that this exercise revealed.

When it had come to contrasting Frank (as I am now) plus his half-sister Holly with Frank Snr, I expected he might say something like 'me and Holly are both young and dad is old', but that wasn't what he said at all.

'Me and Holly are the same because we are related, and my dad isn't.'

I didn't understand. Frank Snr was father to both of them, so this made no sense to me.

'What do you mean, Frank?'

'My dad wants to fight me ….' He took a breath, looking agitated. 'Holly doesn't want to fight me…'

I gave him a moment, sensing he had something significant to say.

'Because Holly is mine.'

'Frank, what do you mean? Holly is yours?'

'Holly is mine,' he repeated. 'She doesn't belong to my dad. Jenny said it, on Bonfire Night.'

I was scribbling our conversation down, word for word, and doing the maths at the same time. My mental arithmetic might not have been as good as his but I worked this one out within a minute. Holly was eight, nearly nine. That meant Frank would have been not yet 14 years old when she was born.

The first person I told was the soft hairy bloke, who turned out to be the unit manager. I did this so the hospital staff could keep a close eye on Frank and offer support if needed.

'Oh, he is a dark horse, isn't he?' the manager laughed. 'Didn't think he'd have it in him.'

After the couple of days I'd had, he was skating on wafer-thin ice. 'Would you have that smile on your face if I'd just told you that a woman in your care had disclosed sexual abuse as a child by her stepfather?' He rearranged his face pretty damn quick, rightly so. Let's make no bones about it, Frank was saying he had been raped by Jenny. She was an adult and he was a child, too young to give consent.

More than a quarter of child sexual-abuse victims are boys. A 2019 YouGov survey for Barnardos showed that more than one in four men find the abuse of teenage boys by women less concerning than the abuse of teenage girls by men. The same survey found that 28 per cent of the adult population thought it was 'every teenage boy's' dream' to be with an older woman. Hopefully the unit manager joined the enlightened 72 per cent after our little discussion.

My next calls, having discussed with Frank what I would be doing, were to his solicitor and then the police, who assured me that they would investigate. As Holly was living at home, they would also make the appropriate referral to social services.

It transpired that it was an open secret within the family that Frank Snr had had a vasectomy long before Holly was conceived. When Jenny fell pregnant everyone in the know – including Frank Snr himself – turned a blind eye to the fact that the child could not have been his.

The real secret may have never come to light if it hadn't been for an innocent remark made by a family member at the Bonfire Night party. One of Frank's young cousins commented on how much Holly looked like him. Given that they were meant to be half-siblings, it was a perfectly reasonable observation to make. But Frank Snr knew they could not be related by blood, or at least he had never considered they could. The cogs must have started turning in Frank Snr's head and he confronted Jenny, telling her she had better come clean or else. 'Is it him?' he yelled, pointing at Frank Jnr.

'Yes, it's him,' Jenny screamed. 'Are you happy now? Are you?'

Nobody was happy. The bomb had exploded in all their faces but it was Frank Jnr who took the biggest hit. Rather than focusing on the appalling fact that Frank had been abused by his stepmother as a young teenager, Frank Snr squared up to Frank Jnr, threatening to kill him. Unsurprisingly, Frank couldn't cope with any of this. He was a child when Holly was conceived. Though Jenny was having sex with him, it had never once occurred to him that it could have resulted in her pregnancy. Scared witless of what might happen next, he ran out of the house.

A few days after I filed my report, Frank was returned to the police station for questioning about the assault on Ian Hayes. My input ended there, but I know he was interviewed for a third time in the presence of his trusty terrier solicitor, who had insisted, after the failings of the first two interviews, that the matter be taken over by a new team of officers. An appropriate adult (as opposed to Frank Snr, the inappropriate adult) was also in attendance, provided by a charity supporting people with autism.

This time, Frank tearfully explained that after Jenny's devastating revelation and his dad's furious response, he wandered the estate, terrified of going home. It was by accident rather than design that he joined the crowds milling around Ian's house that night. And he confessed to the 'murder', and to being a serial killer, because 'I just wanted someone to tell my dad. If I could say I was a killer he would be scared to fight me and people would stop laughing at me.'

What a failure of our culture, I thought to myself, *that a young man like Frank – no matter what his differences – could be inspired at a time of such crisis by our manufactured image of serial killers.* Perhaps he needed to believe that his father was not the most frightening character in the world and that he could be smarter, braver and more worthy of notice if he was more like his perception of those who commit multiple murders. Collectively, serial killers represented his own inner helper, of sorts.

Frank's new story checked out, entirely. No trace of his DNA came back on the analysis of the baseball bat, though Ian's blood and hair were on it, along with the blood of a local hardman. It transpired that Ian had fallen out with this unsavoury character over a dodgy motor deal. He owed the man a considerable amount of money, just as the neighbours had speculated at the start. When the man had come calling, the two argued in the kitchen before Ian picked up the baseball bat he kept handy for such occasions. Unfortunately for Ian, his visitor was the bigger and stronger man. He grabbed the bat and used it to hit Ian round the head before smashing both of his knees in as he tried to run for the door. Ian's hospital visitors had managed to get to him before the police did, which is how he came to know about Frank's handy confession. How convenient it would have been if Ian could have avoided telling the police the truth about his latest illegal business deal, but it was not to be.

When the police eventually tracked down and interviewed the hardman he was wearing trainers that had minuscule specks of Ian's blood soaked into them – airborne droplets that proved he was there at the time of the attack.

To spare their own blushes, the police decided not to charge Frank with perverting the course of justice. He'd found himself in a scary, confusing and dangerous place, and his instinct for self-preservation had been at the root of his false confession.

A paternity test confirmed he was Holly's father and social services began their own investigation. Measures were put in place to safeguard both Frank and Holly, and to help them to navigate their new and complicated family relationships. Ultimately – by a strange and circuitous route – Frank's confession had got him the protection he needed.

CHAPTER FIVE
SNAP DECISIONS

'We have found something quite unexpected, something I think you should take a look at.'

From the pinch-nosed expression on the unit manager's face, I could tell this 'something' was not going to be pleasant. 'I think you're better placed than any of us to shed some light on it. Would you, er, mind?'

When Basil told me what it was, nervously rubbing his thumbs as he did so, I wrinkled my nose a little. 'I'm not a pathologist and I don't like bad smells,' I clarified. 'But go on, then.'

I was working in Laurel House, the same forensic step-down project where, a year later, Nigel would harpoon me with a metal kebab skewer. I'd been providing their psychology service for nearly seven years by this point. It often felt inconvenient to fit in my weekly attendance alongside all the other demands on my time, but working in-depth and meaningfully with the men who lived there was the type of work I loved. And the regular day's work provided me with a sense of continuity among the succession of quick-turnaround assessments.

Basil grabbed his coat and we walked together to the grounds at the back of the main house where the residents were busy building an aviary, a project that had come about after one man brought the budgie he'd kept in prison along with him to the project. It had soon been joined by a parrotfinch called Braveheart (due to his bright blue face markings). On the day of Braveheart's arrival, all the residents started shouting, 'They will never take our freedom!' Suddenly they all wanted a bird of their own. So Basil had scraped some extra money together to create a huge shared aviary to accommodate the expanding winged army.

Several very colourful and chirpy new residents had already arrived. Lined up in a mishmash of large boxes and cages while they waited for the finishing touches to be put on their new abode, they had been keeping an eye on Gordon and Christopher as they dug a trench for a hand-washing station at the rear of the aviary.

Gordon had suffered a personality-altering head injury after falling off the roof of a factory he was breaking into, a cautionary tale if ever there was one. Even at the best of times, he had a tendency to get fixated on things.

'What the hell is that?' he'd suddenly shouted.

His spade had hit something solid, about a foot and a half under the surface.

He and Christopher began clearing away the earth with their bare hands, uncovering a black bin bag that was tied tightly on top.

'What the hell is that!' Gordon shrieked again. 'What the hell is that?' His escalating cries brought another resident and a support worker running and triggered an erratic flurry of activity from the feathered onlookers.

As Gordon and Christopher heaved the bag out of the ground it began to split, emitting a foul smell that knocked them backwards. The other men stood around like undertakers in a cemetery, maintaining a dignified silence while Christopher took a trowel to the bag and teased it open.

'Somebody must be devastated,' Gordon said.

'What do you think?' Basil was now asking me, hanging back while I gingerly took hold of the corner of the potato sack that some thoughtful soul had draped over the top of the open bin bag. *There is only one way to do this*, I thought, taking a deep breath as I pulled the sack back quickly, like I was removing a giant sticking plaster.

Inside the bin bag was the rotting corpse of a small white dog.

A few weeks earlier, I had claimed one of only two desks in the staff office, hoping for some peace and quiet while I typed up my therapy notes. It wasn't to be. The morning was bustling with comings and goings and it wasn't long before a resident came in, his girlfriend in tow. 'You have the seat,' he said to her, indicating the one available chair.

Stuart was a neatly turned-out man in his mid-forties, nondescript in many ways, yet the sort who might be considered to have aged attractively into the silver fox category. The woman – wasp-waisted and slightly younger than him – immediately sat down. As she did so she pulled the two sides of her coat across her body and clasped her hands together.

Stuart hadn't been referred to me but I'd seen him in passing. He was somewhat of an enigma, having unusually moved into the semi-independent annexe, a small house at the back of the project, within weeks of his arrival at Laurel House. The men there weren't under such close supervision as those living in the main building. They enjoyed a few privileges, such as entirely unescorted leave and a budget to do their own grocery shopping and cooking, as they were considered low-risk and tantalizingly close to living their own fully self-sufficient lives. The average stay before a move to the annexe was 12 to 18 months, so I'd sometimes wondered how Stuart had so successfully managed to fast-track himself to a place there.

He had been ushered into the office by the member of staff who was going to sign him out for the day.

'She'll be back in a minute, Lisa,' he said to his girlfriend. 'This won't take long.'

I glanced up from my computer to see him place one hand on the nape of her neck. An innocuous gesture of intimacy, perhaps, but I couldn't help noticing that she flinched, ever so slightly.

'What have you two got planned for today?' I piped up.

Neither of them had acknowledged me sitting there, even though I was only a few feet away from them. I had deliberately directed my question at Lisa but it was Stuart who replied.

'Only going into town to do a bit of shopping,' he said, barely glancing in my direction.

With that, two more residents wedged themselves into the room, followed by the support worker who was signing all three men out for the day. 'It's like Piccadilly Circus in here,' she said to Stuart. 'Come on, let's go through to the back office. There's a bit more space.'

Before any resident left the premises, there was always a form to fill out, detailing where they were going, what they were wearing, how long they would be, who they were with and so on.

Stuart still had his hand resting on his girlfriend's neck.

'You go and wait by the front door,' he instructed her. 'I'll be out in a few minutes.'

I watched as he gave her neck a light squeeze.

As Lisa left the room, tucking her silky brown hair behind her ears as she went, I made a quick decision to find out more about Stuart and their relationship.

I didn't have to wait long. No sooner had I turned my attention back to my computer than the postman arrived at the main entrance. After three rings of the front doorbell it was obvious nobody else was going to answer it so, wondering if I would ever get my admin done for the day, I locked my computer screen and headed for the door. Lisa was standing in the hallway as I signed for the parcel. I gave her a smile and she smiled back, or at least she attempted to. The expression didn't extend to the rest of her face. It was as if someone had pulled two invisible cords at either corner of her mouth and made the edges turn up just enough to give the required illusion.

'Are you looking for anything particular while you are out shopping?' I asked casually, as I closed the door.

She opened her mouth and looked as though she were about to reply but then her eyes flicked over my shoulder.

'Oh, you're very nosy, aren't you?' I heard a man's voice say.

I turned to see Stuart a few paces away, striding towards us. He came and stood between the two of us, his back turned to Lisa and with his face just an inch too close to mine.

He grinned at me, to show that his rhetorical question was merely in jest, but it was the same fabricated smile as his girlfriend's, failing to reach the muscles orbiting his eyes.

'Nosy?' I said, confidently, but feeling compelled to take a step backwards despite myself, to regain my personal space. 'People often say that about me but then I've been called worse. I hope you both have a good day.'

What I really wanted to say was, 'I prefer to call it curiosity, and you can never be too curious in my job,' but I didn't want Stuart to have any hint that he'd just catapulted himself right to the top of my to-do list.

The way a person makes you feel is a highly fickle and fallible source of information. For that reason, I would never draw any conclusions or suggest a course of action based on nothing more than a subjective reaction, or a 'feeling in my waters'. Nevertheless, gut instincts can still be valuable. They are often highly instructive in directing your attention and prompt you to ask further questions that might otherwise have been overlooked.

With all the residents at the unit at potential risk of

reoffending – even those living a hair's breadth away from independence – it was a crucial part of my job to be on the lookout for problems before they happened, with the intention of heading them off at the pass. Even if something felt only slightly or impalpably 'off', I never held back in offering it up for further discussion with my colleagues. It didn't always make me the most popular person in the building but that didn't deter me, my rationale being that it was better to have had the discussion and not needed it than to have needed it and not had it.

'Oh, she is at it again, the mistress of doom!' the staff would sometimes groan as I scanned for holes in a resident's care plan. Either that or they'd hum the Wicked Witch of the West music from *The Wizard of Oz* whenever I said, 'I just want to talk to you about so-and-so...'

The joking (at least I *think* they were joking) was never going to put me off. And certainly not in this case because, in addition to the suspicious and rattled feeling I had around Stuart and his girlfriend, was the fact that, less than five years ago, he had killed the woman he claimed to love.

Before arriving at Laurel House at the end of 2009, he had served half of a seven-year sentence for the manslaughter of his wife Natalie in 2005. They had been married for over ten years and he had claimed to love her, even at the end.

I made a point of finding Basil after I'd finally finished typing up my notes later that afternoon. He was fretting about being late to a meeting and couldn't linger, but I managed to ask him what he made of Stuart.

'Stuart? Er...he's mild-mannered, civil, compliant, the model resident,' he listed, speaking rapidly, as though a buzzer may suddenly sound, cutting him off mid-reply.

'And how do you feel when you spend time with him, would you say?'

Basil considered this for a moment, pouting a little. 'I've not had any issues with him, Kerry. No, none at all. I'm quite at ease with him.'

I considered Basil's answer. He was the type of person who looked for the good in people rather than the bad and I'd always been struck by his ability to be relentlessly positive. His outlook and attitude were impressive in many ways, although perhaps not entirely ideal for somebody running a forensic step-down project full of men who have committed serious offences, where a healthy dose of realism is more the order of the day. Still, Basil was an experienced manager and he cared deeply about getting things right. If he hadn't picked up the same vibes I had about Stuart then I had to consider that maybe I was being overly sensitive, possibly reacting to something that wasn't truly there. I was prepared to accept that and then spend my next clinical supervision meeting working my way through a packet of Hobnobs while trying to figure out if I had 'countertransference' issues ('Is it possible then that you are redirecting the distaste that you feel for that ex-boyfriend, hmm?'). But not before I'd done a bit more homework of my own.

As Basil rushed off, I pulled Stuart's admission notes out of the filing cabinet, which had been assembled in a blue document wallet when he arrived at the unit some six months earlier. The first page told me he had been convicted of the manslaughter of Natalie 'by reason of provocation'.

That old chestnut, I thought to myself.

'Provocation' used to be a partial defence to murder. Under the Homicide Act 1957, in order to be convicted of the lesser charge of manslaughter, and avoid a mandatory life sentence, a defendant would have to satisfy a jury that they were goaded into a temporary loss of all self-control by the words or deeds of another, who was typically their victim.

It is a defence that originates from a time when upper-class men challenged each other to duels when they felt that their 'honour' had been insulted and is steeped in chauvinistic history and clichés. Initially, according to the common law, such outrages as a husband witnessing his wife's adultery or a father discovering a man engaged in what was then considered an 'unnatural act' with his son, constituted provocation. The Act later provided that it could be *anything* that would cause a 'reasonable person' to fly into a passion that left them suddenly no longer the master of their own mind. It is a legal definition that, over the years, has been interpreted liberally in the case of men who kill the women in their lives.

Failing to place a pot of German mustard in the right position on the kitchen table was an apparent affront that cost Thomas Corlett's wife Erika her life in 1985.

'It was her fault. I always placed my newspaper on one side of my plate, the mustard on the other,' the civil servant explained to the police. 'But she moved my paper and put the mustard in its place instead, saying, "That's where I want it, and that's where I will put it."' Not only did the jury at his trial believe that Corlett was sufficiently incited to strangle his wife to death in a fit of ungovernable pique, but the judge expressed sympathy for his plight too, describing him as a 'hard-working man who snapped after skivvying after his wife for years'. Corlett was duly convicted of manslaughter (or 'mans laughter' as writer Julie Bindel suggested was a more appropriate description) by reason of provocation and handed a paltry three-year sentence.

If that outcome wasn't shocking enough, consider the case of Joseph McGrail, who in 1991 killed his partner by kicking her in the stomach while she lay in an alcohol-induced stupor. The judge expressed 'every sympathy' with McGrail, who walked away from court with a two-year suspended sentence. Or Paul Dalton, a teacher who punched his 'domineering' wife Tae Hue Kang so violently that her jaw shattered in two places and then left her to drown in her own blood. He later chopped her body into nine pieces with a chainsaw and hid it in a freezer. During his trial in 2005, he successfully pleaded provocation, claiming that he had 'lashed out in a blind panic' after Tae had taunted him with news of an affair and 'said the most hurtful things'. He was handed a five-year jail term – two years for the manslaughter plus three for preventing the lawful burial of her body.

It's easy to see how provocation – dubbed the 'nagging and shagging defence' by those in legal circles – became the go-to for men accused of killing women (or femicide, as it is now known). The notion of an otherwise psychologically unremarkable man who suddenly 'snaps' and finds himself killing his allegedly hen-pecking, cheating and shrew-like partner while in the 'red mist' (although feel free to insert any number of other disguising euphemisms for homicidal emotions here) proved remarkably resilient, resulting in sympathy and leniency time and time again.

Over the years, several women who have killed their male partners after years of abuse have attempted to claim provocation but with far less favourable results. Being generally less physically strong than men, women typically don't kill without a weapon. And once a woman had reached for a hammer or a knife – or waited for a moment when she was in less direct danger from her abuser – it became nigh on impossible to convince a jury that she had been provoked into a sudden loss of control. Rather, it was easily argued that only a cold-blooded killer would have the presence of mind to take these precautions, not the 'passionate' kind.

Feminist organizations Southall Black Sisters and Justice for Women asserted that provocation was a gendered defence, tailor-made to protect the interests of men who were physically powerful enough to explode into violent anger while throwing women who kill as a result of an accumulation of fear and despair under the proverbial bus. But reforming the law was always going to be like turning around a rusty oil tanker in a silted-up harbour. It took over 20 years of campaigning before, in 2008, proposed changes to the provocation defence were published by Justice Minister Maria Eagle.

By the time I was sitting in a finally peaceful office at Laurel House, with nothing but a ticking clock, the occasional creak of footsteps and the sound of water flushing through the Edwardian plumbing to distract me from Stuart's file, the changes had been accepted. Too late to have impacted in any way whatsoever on his case, they would eventually make their way into law some six months later, in October 2010.

In a nutshell, the reforms meant that 'provocation' was superseded by a somewhat more precisely worded 'loss of control' defence. The crucial difference being that, under the new law, there is no longer a requirement that the loss of self-control be 'sudden', meaning that victims of long-term abuse can cite this as part of a 'qualifying trigger...of an extremely grave character' to the act of killing. In an effort to ensure that men angered by their partner's infidelity no longer get away with murder, it is explicit in stating that cheating in itself cannot be used as a 'qualifying trigger' and juries should ask themselves the question of whether a person in the same circumstances with a 'normal degree of tolerance and control' would have acted the same way.

The reforms were welcome and long overdue, but I couldn't help but muse upon how the real solution required not just a shift in the law, but a far more fundamental shift in our shared attitudes. Will we ever reach a point where a jury faced with the question of whether a 'normal' man vexed by a woman's behaviour might act in the same way will answer, 'No, absolutely not'?

*

Stuart was far from a typical resident at the step-down project. The service was designed for men who needed extensive support. Most were deemed hard to place in other community settings due to their level of risk and severe mental-health challenges, and even for these men it was not easy to secure funding for a bed. Stuart, however, was a qualified accountant and former business owner with no previous history of contact with mental-health services. I would have expected him to have been jettisoned from the prison gates with little more than a grunted goodbye and a future appointment with the probation service, but he had somehow found himself at Laurel House after confiding in a prison officer that he was feeling hopeless about his future upon release.

There were few of the usual interventions required after Stuart walked through the oak and stained-glass door of the step-down project's main house. He was immediately put in touch with an organization that links ex-offenders with job opportunities and had started some part-time work. As an experienced gardener, he also stepped up to organize the relocation of flower beds, shrubs and the project's sizeable vegetable patch. The other men respected his natural authority and it wasn't long before Stuart became the unofficial chief landscaper, a role he took to like a duck to water. He was prescribed antidepressant medication from the in-house psychiatrist and reported no more ups and downs in mood than you would expect of anybody whose life had changed so dramatically from what it once was.

Just a fortnight after he arrived, while accompanied by a discreet support worker, Stuart had met Lisa in a local hardware store, where she was the manager. The relationship progressed quickly, with Stuart 'smitten' – a word used by more than one member of staff in their daily note-keeping – right from the start. After a few weeks of exchanging text messages and enjoying long telephone conversations, he began asking for leave to start dating.

As protocol dictated, a Multi-Agency Public Protection Arrangement (MAPPA) meeting was convened to assess the risks. His offender manager, the probation officer responsible for coordinating his supervision in the community, and a representative from the local police sat with Basil and Stuart's key worker to thrash out the matter. Jointly, they agreed to give Stuart the go-ahead on the condition that Lisa be fully briefed of his circumstances. One important consideration was that the MAPPA panel did not deem Lisa to be a 'vulnerable' woman. She had been in her job for many years and, from what details they had ascertained from Stuart, had a good support network of friends around her. It was clear that she had the capacity to make her own decision about who she wanted to spend time with; all she required was the correct information to base it on.

It came as a surprise to some that, after being given the news that her new love interest was technically still serving time for manslaughter, Lisa didn't immediately flee to the hills. Stuart told Laurel House staff how relieved and 'grateful' he felt when instead she chose to commit to their fledgling romance. By now, their relationship was more than five months old and had progressed to the point where Stuart was allowed to spend one night per week at her home, four miles away. He had told staff that he and Lisa were already talking of a long-term future together.

I imagine that when Lisa was confronted with a choice to make about Stuart, she had done what I was just about to do. Occasionally residents arrive with huge amounts of paperwork but, more often than not, as they travel between institutions, reports are archived and information is lost or condensed into bullet points. Stuart's file was slim, containing an unsatisfying array of dutifully filled-out forms and risk-assessment sheets with too little meat on their bones to reassure me that I understood anything helpful about the man they concerned. So I turned to a more public source of information, tapping his name and Natalie's into a Google search box.

A list of newspaper headlines pinged onto my computer screen. Beneath them was a strip of photographs showing a downcast-looking Stuart against a grey background juxtaposed with a portrait of a smiling blonde woman in a pink bridesmaid's dress. Another photograph showed the pair posing for the camera, tanned and relaxed on holiday. Natalie was pulling a lock of long and shining hair over her top lip like a moustache and kissing the air. Stuart held a bottle of beer in one hand, his head thrown back in laughter. Good times.

I started clicking my way through the press articles. Stuart was described as a 'doting husband' and 'gardening enthusiast' who ran a small courier company. Neighbours told reporters how shocked they were that such a seemingly happy marriage between a 'quiet and private' couple could end in such a terrible way. Natalie's body had been found face down one night on an allotment that the two rented, with injuries to the back of her head similar to those more usually seen in road-accident victims or those who have fallen from a height.

Stuart's barrister had informed the court that his client admitted that he had caused his wife's injuries by first hitting her with a shovel he was holding and then stamping on her. It was 'a short-lived and violent loss of control that was entirely out of character', he said, emphasizing that there was no history of domestic violence between the pair. During sentencing, the judge was quoted as saying Stuart had 'succumbed to a heat-of-the-moment impulse when faced with the realization their relationship was breaking down'. 'You have done something you will regret for the rest of your life,' he remarked as he handed down the sentence, adding, 'It is not lost on me that no punishment that a court can impose can compare with the pain of knowing that, as a consequence of your actions, you have lost the love of your life.' *Why not cook Stuart a casserole as well?* I thought to myself.

If Stuart was the lovesick perpetrator of a *crime passionnel*, Natalie was predictably cast opposite him as the *femme fatale* who had driven him down that path. The judge had bent over backwards to commiserate and the press had been happy to comply with the age-old narrative.

There are recurring themes in the language used in media reporting of male violence against women, a language shared by police, judges, barristers and many others who work in the criminal-justice system. Domestic homicides are recounted as 'tragic events' and 'regrettable incidents'. As the 2020 Femicide Census highlighted, it also 'frequently implies that the victim was somehow responsible for her own death through her actions'. Whether she is described as having a 'chaotic life', being 'difficult to live with', 'using alcohol' or 'beginning a new relationship', the implication is the same: her behaviour did not become her and invited the violence.

I read that Natalie's eye had wandered when her husband's business ran into some financial difficulties. She was 'used to a comfortable lifestyle' and had spent weeks berating Stuart, saying he was a 'terrible provider'. She also criticized his prowess in the bedroom, describing him as a 'useless lover'. On the day of her death, her husband had finally 'snapped' when she had coldly enlightened him that she had found someone else and was leaving him.

Or so Stuart said. It struck me how the story was solely the perpetrator's narrative, unchallenged and now available for all to see online. I wondered if Natalie – the only other witness – would agree that this was an accurate and truthful version of events or feel compelled to stand up and shout, 'No, no, this isn't how it happened.' But dead women can't speak and so Stuart was granted the final word.

By the time Basil returned from his meeting, the sky had turned a spectacular violet and the residents were mostly watching early-evening game shows in the lounge or had dispersed to their respective bedrooms. I could see the shadow of movement in the kitchen of the annexe through the window of the back office.

Basil perched himself on the side of a desk like a Channel 5 newsreader. I let him fill me in about his afternoon before I ventured to ask him how Lisa and Stuart, or rather the relationship between them, was being monitored.

'It's just that I couldn't find anything specified in his care plan or minutes of the MAPPA meetings.'

Basil stood up, then sat back down and re-crossed his legs before getting up again and pulling up a chair, sensing that he had just been softly ambushed.

'Well, I suppose it is informally monitored,' he said. 'We always see them coming and going. Lisa comes here to meet Stuart and so we have plenty of opportunities to speak to her.'

'I've noticed that Stuart's risk assessment wasn't updated when his relationship status changed.'

'Yes, yes, you make a good point,' he said, taking hold of a pad of yellow Post-its. 'I will get on to that.'

'Fantastic. And when you speak to Lisa, do you speak to her alone?'

Basil cleared his throat and told me that no, they did not. Every time a member of staff spoke to Lisa, Stuart was with her.

I raised one eyebrow, the image of his hand on her neck returning to my mind.

Basil nodded sheepishly, then started to tell me, in the vain hope of either reassuring or deflecting me, that Stuart was very attentive to his girlfriend, buying little presents for her all the time. 'He sometimes drops by the hardware shop just to give her some flowers from the garden. It's really quite sweet.'

Or creepy AF, I thought to myself.

'It's clearly an intense relationship,' I said, choosing my words more diplomatically. 'But what passes as romance deserves more consideration in the context of a man who has a history of violence towards women.'

Basil looked positively crushed. 'Don't you think that seems a little harsh, Kerry? Remember, there was no domestic violence in Stuart's marriage until he, um, until, well...'

'He killed his wife,' I added flatly.

'Well, yes, quite,' said Basil.

Domestic abuse doesn't necessarily have to involve violence. Research repeatedly demonstrates that when men kill a current or ex-partner, the fatal act of violence is hardly ever an isolated incident but the endpoint of a sustained period of possessive and controlling behaviours that may or may not include physical assaults and may or may not have been reported to the police. It's a reality that is rarely stated in courtrooms or media reports, the places that have the most influence to shape the public's understanding of femicide. If Stuart was an exception to that rule, he was a unicorn indeed.

Basil was leaning forward, fiddling defensively with the Post-its. 'Stuart and I have spoken about his offence and he is deeply remorseful. He fully admits that the red mist descended.'

'Do you really believe in red mist?' I sighed.

'Don't you?'

'No, I don't. I believe that violence is a choice that people make when they are in a position of power over someone else. Granted, some people have more choices than others. I'm usually the first to point that out. But there is always a choice.'

Basil nodded respectfully, a thoughtful expression on his face.

The killing of women and girls by men is a global problem of epidemic proportions. Violence against women is more prevalent in societies that ascribe greater status to men than to women, just as it is in those cultures that place high emphasis on family honour and sexual purity, or where male entitlement is sanctioned and accepted at the expense of women's rights. But even westernized cultures are not nearly as female-friendly as you might expect. The Femicide Census data show that in the ten years from 2009 to the end of 2018, at least 1,425 women were killed by men in England, Wales and Northern Ireland. Or to put it another way, one woman was killed every three days, and this number is starting to rise. Men who were in an intimate relationship with the victim, or had been, were responsible for 62 per cent of these deaths.

'I may have formed an undeservedly negative impression of Stuart,' I went on, 'but there is one thing I'm sure of.'

'What's that?' asked Basil.

'When he killed Natalie, it wasn't because he had *lost* control. It was because he wanted to *exert* control.'

When I arrived for my shift two weeks later, Basil sprang out of his office to tell me he'd spoken to Lisa himself, on her own.

'How did it go?'

'Absolutely fine. She said everything was absolutely fine. No problems whatsoever.'

'What did she say?'

'She said Stuart is still keen. And he has high hopes for their future together, which sounds encouraging.'

'And Lisa? What does she want from the relationship?'

'She said she'd expected them to take things a little bit slower. It's the first relationship she's been in for several years, since her divorce, but she said she had got used to it and everything is going well.'

I didn't want to burst Basil's bubble but he'd gleaned precisely nothing from Lisa.

'Where did you talk to her?'

'Right here,' he said, gesturing towards his office. 'Stuart took himself out into the garden to help unload the aviary materials and there was nobody else around, so there were no distractions whatsoever…'

It seemed wholly inadequate to me. The issue was not whether there were any 'distractions' but whether Lisa was in a situation where she felt able to speak freely. With Stuart just a stone's throw away and fully aware of what was taking place, was she really going to feel able to open up? And to the male unit manager?

When I put this gently to Basil he looked exasperated, his sucked-in cheeks indicating that my mistress-of-doom reputation had struck again, although he was too polite to shut me down.

'Right,' he said, rolling out the word a little too long to sound persuaded, 'what do you suggest?'

I suggested that a full-time female member of staff – perhaps Maggie – should telephone Lisa one evening when Stuart was busy cooking his dinner and fix up a meeting somewhere neutral. Maggie was an observant support worker who was easy to talk to and had worked at the project seemingly forever. Basil agreed, retreating back into his office and closing the door before I could insert myself, uninvited, into another model resident's business.

There was a locked archive cupboard in one of the offices at the project, where any miscellaneous bits of paper were stored for the duration of a resident's stay with us. In the past, it had proved to be a diamond mine, throwing up precious gems of information such as full parole-board dossiers and court depositions that shone a sometimes dazzling light on a resident's story. I hadn't yet found the moment to mention it to Basil but I'd emailed the project's part-time secretary to ask her if she would dig anything relating to Stuart out of the cupboard for me. My request yielded a smattering of old papers from his time in prison, telling me that he had held a trusted position as a cleaner on B wing and had completed a plastering course. There were also some forms from when he was serving time on remand, prior to his conviction, and was being monitored for possible self-harm or suicide. A handwritten account of a conversation that he had had with a prison officer at this time, though hard to decipher, proved interesting.

Stuart had let slip that, when the police first knocked on his door and informed him of the discovery of his wife's body, he had claimed no knowledge of what had befallen her. Instead, he insisted that he had been at home all evening, concerned that Natalie hadn't returned any of his calls. He invited the policeman to check his car, a fleet vehicle from his courier company that was fitted with a device that logged all journeys taken. It had been sitting in his driveway since lunchtime.

It was only when Stuart was confronted with physical evidence placing him at the scene of Natalie's death and statements of witnesses who had seen him walking the 90-minute round trip between the marital home and the allotment where she was found that he made a confession.

Stuart may enjoy a good walk but it seemed a strange coincidence that he would leave his car, complete with its GPS technology, on the drive on that particular day.

'I'm worried that it won't play well in court,' he had told the prison officer.

He needn't have worried, as it seems that the prosecution didn't mention it as part of their case at all.

Basil phoned me at home on a damp spring morning, a few days after he'd led me to the grounds to take a look at what the men had unearthed while working on the aviary.

'What's your opinion?' he had asked me while we were kneeling over the dog's body.

'Well, I'm no vet but it is definitely dead,' I said facetiously, while privately thinking about my cat Bijou and what an integral and irreplaceable part of the family all of my childhood pets had been.

The dog had definitely been someone's pet. It was still wearing a turquoise padded harness with a reflective trim, proof that somebody had cared enough to worry that it could be seen properly on night walks. But there was no collar or identity tag.

I told Basil that, by the size and shape of it, I guessed it might have been a bichon frisé type of cross-breed, but I couldn't be sure. Its face was blackened and pointed but there was plenty of crinkly white fur clinging to the skin, so I imagined it couldn't have been in the ground for very long.

'How long, do you think?'

'I really don't know. I suppose it depends on how deep it has been buried and the climate. All I can say is that it is definitely fresh enough for you to be concerned about how it got here.'

I couldn't see any obvious cause of death – no tyre marks or implement sticking out of its body – but the dog was curled into a ball, its underside stuck to the bin bag it was found in. Not being a canine crime scene investigator or wanting to look too closely, my limited insight was now exhausted.

'Let's get it to a vet and see if it's microchipped,' I said.

Since his grim discovery, Gordon had been able to talk of nothing else. He was convinced the dog had been the victim of a hit and run (and had then presumably buried itself). He had also had to be talked down from standing on the main road in front of the project, pointing a broken electric drill at passing traffic, pretending it was a speed gun. Not to mention that the other residents were starting to lose patience with how many times he said, 'Somebody's going to be devastated.'

I had been scoring up some psychometrics when Basil called me at home. He didn't normally phone me on the days I wasn't at the project. I asked what I could help him with.

'Ah. We've heard from the vets and I thought it best to share the news.'

'Go on.'

I could tell from the hesitant tone in his voice that something was wrong.

'Well, under the circumstances, I thought it best to ask the vet if they could provide any information about how the animal died. So they are going to take a look and let me know their findings later. Obviously they have to prioritize their other, living patients as it is quite an unusual request.'

His extended preliminaries were making me even more intrigued.

'I understand. But was it microchipped?'

I heard Basil exhale.

'It was. He was eight years old and his name was Chewy. And, I'm afraid to tell you, he belonged to Stuart's girlfriend.'

Lisa was very surprised to see us standing on her doorstep later that day. After some debate, Basil and I had decided on the most discreet course of action. We went to her home unannounced, early in the evening when we knew Stuart was tucked away in his flat and had no plans to see Lisa the following day.

After doing a double take, the colour immediately drained from Lisa's face.

'Has something happened to Stuart? Has he done something to himself?'

'No, no, he's perfectly fine,' Basil reassured her. 'We would just like to talk to you about another matter, if we may?'

Lisa showed us into her living room, a bit of colour already returning to her cheeks. I was grateful to have Basil at my side. Although, as usual, he was being overly self-conscious, fussily offering to take his shoes off and making an unnecessary song and dance over which chair he should sit in, he was a gentle presence and I could tell he helped ease this intrusion into Lisa's night.

We had agreed that I would be the one to deliver the bad news, sticking only to the facts, of course, and being careful not to make any accusations.

I started with the news that Chewy had been found dead. This obviously came as a shock to her, as Lisa looked stricken.

'Where?' she spluttered, though she must have already had a clue this was going to be something she didn't want to hear.

When I told her it was in the grounds of Laurel House, one hand shot to her mouth and the other clutched at her stomach.

'I don't understand.'

She started looking around the room, as if searching for answers, but was somehow not looking at anything. 'But how? Oh my God! He knew I loved that dog…'

Once Lisa had taken a moment to let the information sink in, she managed to tell us that her pet had gone missing some two months previously. She presumed he had escaped from the garden and had spent hours putting up missing posters all over the neighbourhood, helped on occasion by Stuart. 'I was so upset and he said he didn't like to see me like that. He said he would do whatever it took to help bring Chewy home.'

She was gasping in disbelief now, as if hit by a fresh wave of realization, and she was repeating herself as she tried to take it in, 'He helped me. He said he would do whatever it took...'

There was a newly printed batch of posters on the sideboard, which Lisa drew our attention to. 'I hadn't given up hope of finding him. He was microchipped, you see... Are you sure? Are you absolutely sure it's him?'

It was a desperate question and she only had to look at our faces to know the answer.

'What happened to him? How did he die?'

The vet had ruled out any road traffic accident. Instead, he had pointed to what he called a 'blunt force head trauma', explaining that Chewy had suffered a blow to the head that was so hard that he had suffered a 'contrecoup injury', which is severe bruising to the opposite side of the brain to where the impact occurred. How exactly it had been caused was a mystery.

'We don't know the circumstances of how he died,' I said. 'At the moment, all we know is that the vet we took him to said that he had an injury to his head. We would very much like to know as well and so if there's anything you can tell us that might help, please do.'

She stared at the jute rug under her feet. 'He did it. It had to be Stuart, didn't it?'

'I can't say that,' I said, telling her that though Stuart was aware a dog had been found in the grounds, he hadn't been made aware of any other developments. 'But I'm interested to know why you would think that,' I added.

Lisa lapsed into silence.

Basil offered to go and wait in the car, to 'leave you ladies alone if that would help to make things easier'. But Lisa entreated him to stay and their mutual embarrassment prompted her to admit that, 'Silly as it sounds, Stuart seemed jealous of Chewy at times. He said I gave him too much attention. But then after I lost him, he told me we could get another dog one day. One that belonged to both of us. He would train it, he said.'

'Is there anything else about Stuart's behaviour towards Chewy, or yourself, that makes you feel he might have wanted to harm him?'

'It's hard for me, because I'm…' There was a pause before she pushed herself to finish her sentence. 'Because I'm scared. I'm scared to say.'

'Scared?'

'Yes. Because…' There was another pause. 'Because he's told me he can't live without me. He will kill himself if he loses me.'

She dropped back into her chair, as if some tension had left her body along with this disclosure.

'I feel so stupid. All of my friends warned me not to get involved. But I gave him the benefit of the doubt. He told me that his wife had cheated on him when his business was in trouble, that he had loved her so much that he had some sort of breakdown. The newspapers said it was true, he was a good husband, a decent bloke who had just flipped. I suppose I felt sorry for him.'

I noticed Basil's shoulders shifting a little closer to his ears out of my peripheral vision. *Stuart does have considerable talent for eliciting sympathy*, I thought.

Lisa went on, admitting that the disapproval of her family and friends caused her to back off from them. Meanwhile, Stuart told her that she didn't need people in her life who didn't want her to be happy. He showered her with gifts and compliments. He talked about their future together, even though she started to feel uncomfortable and asked him to slow down. 'When I raised it with him, he got upset. He said I was ungrateful. And that, after everything he had been through, I was the only thing in life worth carrying on for.'

'That's a huge amount of emotional pressure to be under,' I commented, 'but Stuart's welfare is our responsibility while he is at Laurel House. It can't be yours.'

'I've been working up the courage to tell Maggie,' she nodded. 'But I was scared that he would be livid with me if I did.'

'Are you frightened of him?' Basil asked.

Lisa looked up at us both with an expression that said it all. When your partner has already proved himself capable of killing one woman, can there be any clearer intimation, even if never said out loud, that if you step out of line, you might be next?

'Can I show you something?'

We followed Lisa through a small dining room into a square kitchen at the back of the house. She stopped in front of a wooden stand sitting on the laminate floor with two stainless-steel dog bowls inside it, waiting optimistically for Chewy's return. Basil and I gazed at her expectantly, not quite understanding the significance of why we were gathered there.

Lisa pointed to the wall.

Stuck fast to the ivory-painted plaster was a black Nokia mobile telephone. Stuart had taken out a contract on it, she said, despite her owning a mobile already. One night when he was staying over, he had asked her to bring a heavy-duty adhesive from the shop she managed and he had fixed it in place. Now he could be certain she was definitely at home whenever he called her in the evenings.

'Sometimes he phones or texts six or seven times in the night. I've asked him not to. It wakes me up and I have to come downstairs to answer his calls, or he accuses me of being with my friends or even another man. If I ignore a call, he will question me about it for hours. It's not worth it; I don't sleep now and just do what he wants. But I don't know how much longer I can go on for.'

When we left the house an hour later, it was difficult to judge who was more dumbfounded by the day's revelations – Lisa or Basil.

'I'd like to address the fact that I owe you an apology, Kerry,' he said, after he had arranged his long limbs behind the wheel of his car and double-checked I was wearing my seat-belt.

'Don't be silly,' I told him. 'You don't owe me anything. You were seduced.'

And not just by Stuart, I thought to myself, *but by the myth of men who 'snap' and all of the institutionalized misogyny that surrounds and perpetuates it.*

We had given Lisa our repeated assurance that our paramount concern was for her and Stuart's safety. Maggie would be in touch with her tomorrow to chat through how she was feeling and she was left in no doubt she could rely on our support, whatever it was she chose to do next.

'Perhaps there is a good explanation for what happened to Chewy,' she had said before we left her house, more to herself than anybody else.

'Perhaps,' I'd responded. 'Although there is no justification for the fear that you've been living in.'

'I've got a lot of thinking to do, haven't I?'

'You do. Perhaps give one of those friends you have been avoiding a call. I'm sure that they will be relieved to hear from you.'

I had a feeling that it wasn't just Lisa's friends who were going to play a part in helping her to gain some perspective of the situation she had found herself in. Basil had scheduled a telephone meeting first thing in the morning with Stuart's offender manager.

It was the offender manager, accompanied by a police officer, who spoke to Stuart about the dog. Without missing a beat, Stuart claimed he had found it in the street outside Lisa's house, having been hit by a car. To spare her pain, he brought it back to the unit and gave it a 'decent send-off'.

An implausible story, even without the vet's report, but one Stuart would stick to. However, he didn't have such a ready explanation up his sleeve for when he was asked about the mobile phone glued to his girlfriend's wall. The indignant surprise that particular line of questioning brought about was only surpassed by the shock that apparently registered on his face the moment he was informed that he was being recalled to prison. He was to serve the three-year remainder of his sentence and was therefore duly arrested on the spot.

A person can be recalled to prison for breaking the conditions of their licence, committing a further offence or, as was officially the case with Stuart, behaving in such a way as to cause their supervisor to believe that they were on the brink of committing a crime. An alternative may have been a 'supervised break-up', with the forensic step-down staff and Stuart's offender manager working together to ensure Lisa's safe exit from the relationship, if that's what she wanted. But, to my mind, the right decision had been taken. Chewy hadn't fared so well, but Lisa was undoubtedly a survivor of 'coercive control', a pattern of behaviours that wasn't recognized as criminal in the UK until December 2015.

The Femicide Census found that almost 40 per cent of women killed by men had first been subjected to coercive control, a statistic that proves that the more well-known warning signs – escalating assaults (particularly if they involve strangulation) and injury – are far from the only indicators a woman is at risk of meeting a violent end.

Perpetrators of coercive control deploy a range of tactics to influence, intimidate, threaten, isolate and surveil their victim. The aim is to exert and sustain their dominance over another person, chipping away at their independence until they dance to the tune of their abuser, trapped and manipulated like a puppet on a string. It is when a perpetrator fears losing this power that they resort to physical violence to regain control. Controlling men are never more fearful than when a woman challenges their status or asserts herself enough to leave the relationship. It is then that their thinking shifts from '*She can't do this to me; I can't live without her*' to '*I won't let her do this to me; she won't live if it's without me.*'

When it is not accompanied by black eyes and broken bones, coercive control can be difficult to spot, particularly when the shame and fear that prevent victims from reporting what they are going through are helped along by the sexist tropes held up by the popular press and the justice system. There are many signs that predict when a woman is in danger, but we are just not trained to recognize or act on them – or, worse still, we are conditioned to excuse them.

In her book *In Control: Dangerous Relationships and How They End in Murder*, criminologist Professor Jane Monckton Smith details the eight-stage model – based on analysis of 372 cases of men who killed their wives or girlfriends – that reveals the typical 'homicide timeline', or chronology of events. In a blow to the 'moment of madness' narrative, stage seven is the planning stage. In many of the cases, the research found evidence of premeditation, in the form of purchasing weapons, internet searches for methods of killing, digging graves or perhaps preparing an alibi. Proof of the fallacy that men kill women in crimes of passion. They do not. Men kill women in crimes of *possession*.

Mistress of doom? A nosey parker? All part of the job description as far as I'm concerned. Paying more attention never killed anyone but it could save a life. Lisa told us she had been working up the courage to tell Maggie about some of Stuart's behaviour. So had the discovery of poor Chewy not thrown a spanner into Stuart's works as it did, I'd like to think that the measures we had (eventually) put in place to safeguard Lisa would have allowed her to share what was happening to her before it was too late. But the case still reinforced a valuable lesson. Domestic abusers can be likeable and attractive and are adept at appealing to our better nature. But if we make it our business to look closer and are prepared to recognize more than bruises and broken bones as indicators of life-threatening abuse, fewer women will die at the hands of men.

CHAPTER SIX
AN EMPTY ROOM

I was eating my breakfast as I sifted through the morning post. The letter on top of the pile looked as innocuous as the handful of others that came that day. A bland, white A4 envelope, franked not stamped. The sort I get all the time, hopefully containing notification that one of my invoices had at last been paid or, more likely, some legal documents I'd requested.

I took a sip of tea and opened it.

It was from a solicitor. No surprise there. Plenty of my correspondence comes from solicitors, though I'd never dealt with this particular one before. I scanned the first paragraph. Would I be available to carry out a pre-sentence assessment of his client? I raised an eyebrow. Usually a request like this would come during an initial phone call. There were also several sheets attached, even though normally I'd only be sent the paperwork once I'd agreed to take the job on.

I casually turned over the covering letter while simultaneously helping myself to a mouthful of Fruit 'n Fibre.

'What the…?'

In front of me was a photocopy of a close-up photograph of a crime scene. I grimaced and instinctively put two fingers to my lips, as if to stop my breakfast escaping.

It's not unusual to feel your stomach lurch when you see a crime scene photo for the first time. It goes with the territory and you get used to it, to a certain extent. You know to steel yourself when one is coming your way, but even so it has a visceral effect. Scene-of-crime videos are the same. The first time you watch, you're simultaneously recoiling and trying to take in the overall story while you wait for your adrenaline to subside. On your next viewing, your automatic physiological response has calmed down, allowing you to take in the details and make notes.

This photograph was hardly up there with some of the most gut-churning I'd ever seen in over 15 years in this career by that point but still, I was appalled. What kind of ghoulish character sends this without calling first? I needed fair warning, if indeed I needed to see it at all, and how presumptuous to assume I would agree to the work? I was also feeling bloody angry on behalf of the woman in the image.

Her name was Mairead, I read.

What would Mairead have thought about this undignified image being delivered to a stranger's breakfast table along with the gas bill and a pile of junk mail?

Death is an incredibly intimate event. Some people believe that once someone is dead, they're long past caring what they look like and what happens to them, but I don't agree. It's enough to irk me when a friend puts up a picture of me on Facebook taken at an unflattering, three-chins angle or mid-snort. Not only because I'm vain and I don't want to be seen looking like something that lives under a bridge and scares small children, but because I find it disrespectful to share another person's image without asking first.

Dead people are people nonetheless. And when you're dealing with a person who has died, I think you need to show an even greater level of respect because they are not able to stamp their foot and demand the same consideration as their neighbour. And trust me, this unfortunate woman would not have wanted to be seen this way by anybody at all.

It was too late to look away. I couldn't un-see this image and professional curiosity began to replace my initial shock and annoyance as I took in the details of the photograph.

Mairead was lying in bed, her body covered up to the curled twigs of her shoulders by a duvet with pretty gingham hearts on it. A heavily stained sheet was turned back over the top of the duvet. The sheet must have been covering Mairead's face initially, I realized: the yellow-brown patches on it were the residue of decomposed skin that had been peeled away when the sheet was turned back.

What was left of Mairead's face had taken on the appearance of dark melted wax. Her features were not instantly recognizable as the components of a human face, though her incongruously white upper dentures were still in the cavern of her mouth, lolling at a slightly jaunty angle.

Grey hairs formed a haphazard semi-circle around the top of Mairead's head and were stuck fast to the discoloured pillow. Piled around the edges of the pillow were lots of white plastic air fresheners – the sort you get in pound shops and look like small cages filled with multi-coloured jelly crystals.

Dotted among them were little bottles of holy water, shaped like the Virgin Mary, that you might buy from a tourist stall outside the Vatican or at Lourdes. It would take a lot more than a trip to Lourdes to revive this poor soul, I thought.

At the side of Mairead's shoulder lay a magazine and I could just make out a fat black fly, sitting on one of the curling corners.

I returned to the paperwork, wanting to know more.

Mairead was a retired nursery nurse in her seventies. Her body had been discovered in her bedroom, in the back of the bungalow she shared with her younger sister, Evelyn, who was in her late fifties.

Evelyn was the solicitor's client. She had been charged with 'preventing the lawful and decent burial of a corpse', the maximum sentence for which is life imprisonment.

The word 'decent' struck me. How we treat dead bodies is incredibly important, as reflected in the maximum sentence. Our basic human instinct to revere the dead is exactly why I'd reacted so negatively to the unsolicited image. In our culture, we afford the dead great privacy, removing them to a chapel of rest and only allowing loved ones to visit, to say a last goodbye. Even then, many people choose not to go, preferring to remember the person as they were in life rather than death.

Not all cultures behave this way. Take Indonesia's Toraja people. They treat the dead as merely sick, offering them food and drink and even cigarettes on a daily basis, believing that the spirit remains near the body and craves care during the period of 'transition' to the afterlife. The ritual may go on for months or even years – the body preserved with formalin – until the family has saved enough money for a suitable funeral. Death is merely one step in a long, unfolding journey.

Unfortunately for Evelyn, she lived in an industrial town in Lancashire, not among the Toraja people of Indonesia. And now she was facing a very serious charge.

I wondered how long Mairead's corpse had lain decomposing under her gingham-hearts duvet before she was discovered. How had she died and why had her sister left her for so long?

Preventing the lawful and decent burial of a corpse is a rare charge, one I'd never dealt with before (or since). Often it's related to other crimes, sometimes very serious ones.

There was a heartbreaking case in 2013, when mother-of-eight Amanda Hutton was found guilty of the charge after concealing the body of her four-and-a-half-year-old son, Hamzah Khan, for nearly two years. The little boy's mummified body was discovered in a travel cot in a bedroom strewn with rubbish. He'd died of severe malnutrition and Hutton had hidden his death to cover up her abuse – she was also convicted of gross-negligence manslaughter and child neglect.

The following year, serial killer Joanna Dennehy and two accomplices were convicted of preventing the lawful and decent burial of men she had murdered. One of them, Kevin Lee, a married father of two, was left in a roadside ditch dressed in a black sequin dress and with his buttocks exposed. The prosecution said the way in which his body was dumped was 'deliberately engineered as an act of post-death humiliation'.

Perhaps the most intriguing case – at least from a forensic psychologist's viewpoint – is that involving the Tetra Pak heir Hans Kristian Rausing. He was convicted of preventing the lawful and decent burial of his wife Eva, who had died of heart failure while the couple were in the grip of drug addiction. He had hidden her body for two months under a pile of clothes in the single room they'd been living in at their mansion home. 'I know it sounds selfish, but I just didn't want her to leave,' he told a psychiatrist.

Though the motives in those three cases are varied – covering up the death of a child, feeding the kicks of a serial killer and the desperate desire to keep a loved one close – there is a common thread. They are all stories on top of stories. The prevention of a decent burial is an addendum to a harrowing and catastrophic sequence of events.

So what was Evelyn's backstory?

The letter told me she was also charged with benefit fraud, after collecting Mairead's weekly pension payments from the post office. Not such a rare charge but interesting when linked to the first. That said, I didn't imagine financial gain was what drove Evelyn. Cashing in a state pension isn't exactly the Great Train Robbery, is it? Judging from the photograph, no particular effort had been made to hide her sister's body, so it was inevitable that she was going to be discovered at some point, exposing the pension fraud easily.

Evelyn intended to plead guilty to both charges and the solicitor wanted to present her psychological assessment to the court in mitigation prior to sentencing.

There was a brief psychiatrist's report attached to the letter. A 'mental state examination' had been carried out but it gave little away. It provided the psychiatrist's observations of Evelyn's appearance, emotions and behaviour on the day of her assessment, but all this snapshot really proved was that she had got dressed that morning, made good eye contact and did not appear to be hallucinating. Her mood was (not surprisingly) 'low'; she was described as 'feeling guilty' and the report concluded she was suffering from a 'moderate depressive disorder' and required antidepressant medication, the modern-day panacea.

Ordinarily, if they are not living at Her Majesty's pleasure or in a hospital, I see forensic clients at their solicitor's office, for practical or safety reasons. But the solicitor requested that I carry out my assessment at his client's home – the bungalow where Mairead's corpse was found. Something about the bold font told me that it was an order rather than a request.

We've got a right one here, I thought, cursing him all over again. Why send me to the house where a dead body had been stashed in the back bedroom?

I thought back to the urban legend of the man in New Mexico who encased the embalmed body of his wife in a glass coffee table. A totally implausible tale, not least because the story appeared in the *Weekly World News*, an entertainment tabloid well known for its preposterous headlines, complete with a photograph in which the 'coffee table' looked suspiciously like a large fish tank turned on its side. For a moment my imagination ran wild. If Evelyn stored a dead body in the bedroom, what else might she have lying about the place? Her old pet cat down the back of the sofa? I checked myself and read on.

Mairead had been discovered in quite a typical way in such circumstances: neighbours had made several complaints to her landlord about mice, flies and a foul odour coming from the property. The landlord had called the police after going round to investigate and finding the flies congregating all over the back bedroom window. When confronted, Evelyn had immediately told police that Mairead's body was in the room and gave the date of her death as some nine weeks earlier. *Nine weeks.*

Inconsiderate solicitor or not, I wanted to take on the case. I wanted to know everything about Evelyn's mindset and what made her leave her sister's body rotting in the back bedroom for all that time. Of course I did. There it was again – oddity, particularly psychological oddity, has always had an irresistible allure for me.

On the morning of my appointment to visit Evelyn, I started to wonder what I'd let myself in for, not least in terms of what possible biohazards might be awaiting me.

Nine weeks was a long time for a body to languish in a back bedroom. It had been over the summer, too. While it had been a typically disappointing British summer, a body left to its own devices for more than two months in any weather is going to turn the air rancid and potentially attract a lot more than a swarm of flies. I stood in front of my wardrobe, thinking about what to wear for the visit.

Half-wincing at the memory, I thought about a highly strung clinical psychologist called Judith whom I worked with years earlier, when I was a trainee. What would she have worn if she were in my shoes? The question amused me.

Judith had gone into a decline when she was allocated an out-patient whose notes mentioned she had had recurrent fleas.

'I'm going to need a plan!' Judith had cried, clearly very agitated.

I found it funny. You don't go into forensic psychology and not expect to come across the occasional client who's carrying round a few little visitors. I'm not suggesting that the people I work with are necessarily any less hygienic than anybody else, but occasionally personal grooming can take a dip when a person lives in extreme poverty or is defeated by the effort of simply staying afloat.

I've seen the odd flea hop across the table when I'm talking to a patient. My response is to calmly crunch the little sucker with the tip of my pen, giving me the same feeling of satisfaction as popping bubble wrap. I've also encountered a number of lice in my time. Once I watched a whole family of them fall out of the unusually thick eyelashes of a male client and, memorably, I witnessed prison inmates attempting to race pubic lice. That's how bored you can get in prison.

You also get the occasional whiffy patient.

'Peter's wearing his "Cabbage Pour Homme",' we used to say in one hospital. Or 'Mandy has her "Eau de Toilet" on today.' And then we'd have a conversation about which member of staff was best placed to broach the delicate subject of body odour with the person concerned, who was already likely to be struggling.

Judith, however, was not the kind to recognize that the problem was a lot more uncomfortable for the patient than it was ever going to be for her. No. Judith was going to do everything in her power to protect herself from the threat of a few fleas. For a start, she was going to choose an outfit that covered every inch of her skin, she decided. She would also roll up the carpet in her office and pile up everything bar two chairs at the far end of the room. Then immediately after the appointment, she was going to sprint to the shower.

I realized that to get to the staff bathroom she'd have to dash from the reception area past the secretaries' offices. I wanted to see what outfit she'd plumped for, so when the appointment was due to end I loitered in one of the offices, from where I'd be able to catch a glimpse of the Judith show.

When the moment came and she appeared, legging it down the corridor, I couldn't believe my eyes.

The lengths she'd gone to were astonishing. Judith was wearing what can only be described as a disposable hazmat suit, the legs of which were tucked into thick socks and a pair of lace-up boots. Her long hair was scraped into a tight bun, secured by shower cap. She looked more like a chemical-weapons expert tackling some kind of nuclear fallout than a clinical psychologist dealing with a patient who might have a few pesky passengers on board. Did she think the fleas would be radioactive?

I was flabbergasted, and so was Judith's patient. Such was the layout and exit system of the hospital, the woman was still standing in the air lock in the reception area, waiting to be let out, when Judith sprinted past. I met her gaze just as we were both caught in the same wide-eyed 'what the fuck?' expression. She shook her head and I shrugged apologetically.

Way to go to build up therapeutic rapport, Judith, I thought.

I was never going to go that far but, all the same, I opted to wear a sturdy pair of knickers on the day I went to Evelyn's bungalow. I had no idea what state the house would be in. For all I knew, it could be shining like a new pin but, just to be on the safe side, Bridget Jones pants seemed like a sensible choice, in case some critter decided to scamper up my trouser leg when I sat on the sofa.

Driving there, I started imagining what sort of person Evelyn was. There's no set assessment procedure to follow in these circumstances but I'd be spending around three hours in her company, talking to her, asking questions and taking notes in order to write up my report. How had she lived with the knowledge that her sister's body was rotting in the back bedroom week after week? As I turned into her street, I noticed my top lip curling.

Evelyn lived on a small, well-kept estate made up of a mixture of council and privately owned houses. I spotted the bungalow at the end of a crescent and for a split second I imagined I saw a large coffin, not a small home.

Evelyn's was the only property still with the curtains drawn at 11.30am, but otherwise the house was very ordinary looking, giving no clue as to the grim secret it had harboured that summer. As I parked up, I took in the small front garden, which was neat and tidy and stocked with as many ornaments as shrubs – cherubs and woodland creatures made of stone and garden gnomes grinning brightly, holding fishing rods and watering cans.

I rang the bell. When Evelyn answered the door I felt an instant pang of guilt – I don't know how I imagined she would look but it wasn't like this. I shouldn't allow myself any preconceived ideas but clearly I had, albeit subconsciously. Mentally, I kicked myself.

Evelyn was a woman who took a lot of pride in her appearance. Her grey-blonde hair was blow-dried into a neat bob; she was dressed in a fashionable yellow blouse and was perfectly made-up. She was very welcoming too, smiling and thanking me for 'coming over', as if I were a friend dropping in for coffee.

I caught a waft of her sweet-smelling perfume as I followed her inside – then I immediately felt the hot illuminating glow of a 100-watt lightbulb turning on in my brain. I gave a silent nod to the solicitor, who had suddenly gone up massively in my estimation.

No wonder he wanted the assessment carried out in Evelyn's home, I thought. He was absolutely right to arrange it this way because clearly the bungalow itself was going to tell me a great deal about its inhabitant. Despite having only just crossed the doorstep, it was already obvious that Evelyn had a considerable problem, one that was no doubt very pertinent to the serious charge she was facing.

'Come through,' she said in her strong Northern Irish accent, steering me into the lounge. 'Here we are now.'

I tried not to show it on my face but I'd never seen anything like it.

The room was piled high with clutter, everywhere you looked. Like a bric-a-brac store had vomited, several times over. I knew from the psychiatric report that Evelyn worked part-time in a clothes-alteration shop and there was fabric everywhere, stacked in precarious-looking heaps. And all around were ornaments, boxes of magazines and papers, framed pictures and books, plant pots and plastic coat hangers, stacked up high. And when I say high, I mean five-foot tall towers of chaos.

'I'll take you through to my sister's bedroom and I can show you her report.'

Evelyn didn't acknowledge the mess but I could tell she was trying to steer me through it as quickly as possible.

I was trying not to goggle but I felt like my eyes were on stalks. More books, knitting patterns and bags of wool, bulging plastic bags, vinyl records, clothes, several lamp stands with no shades, a broken shelf unit, Christmas decorations.

An ammonia smell caught the back of my throat and started to make my eyes sting. Was it mouse or rat pee, maybe?

There was a sofa buried under the clutter but there was no danger I'd have to sit on it as I'd feared – you could scarcely make it out. The only piece of furniture not covered in debris was a leather armchair which pointed towards the TV, the thinnest corridor of clear space between the two.

'Come this way, come on.'

Evelyn was leading me through a narrow tunnel. I followed her, the teetering piles on either side reaching up to my shoulders and almost up to her ears.

Emerging out of the back of the living room, I caught a glimpse of the small kitchen. The sink looked just about accessible but the cooker was almost completely hidden behind food boxes, jars, cans, brushes, brooms and plastic bags. Empty bottles, buckets and cardboard boxes bulging with cloths, newspapers and all kinds of gadgets littered the floor.

There were lots of questions I wanted to ask, but all in good time. I followed Evelyn's lead.

We crossed a tiny internal hallway and squeezed past the bathroom. I glanced in. There was a clear run to the loo and sink – both perfectly clean-looking – but the rest of the floor and all the surfaces were heaped with lotions and potions and a mishmash of towels, clothes and toiletries.

Mairead's bedroom was at the very back of the bungalow. As we entered it, the ammonia smell that was burning my eyes was replaced by a pungent, sickly cocktail. It's hard to describe it. They say the smell of death sticks to you and it certainly felt like that. It was heady, unavoidable, invasive. The bedroom window was ajar, letting in a cool draught, but that wasn't helping much. I couldn't stop my nose from wrinkling and had to hold my breath for a moment in order to deal with the stench, while Evelyn seemed completely oblivious to it.

I gave a mental salute in solidarity with the police who'd been first on the scene and the hapless team from environmental health who had come to clean up after the corpse was taken away. What a job they'd had.

The bedroom was now empty save for fitted wardrobes, a two-foot-high stack of paperwork in the corner – which looked ready to take root and grow like ivy – plus two fold-up chairs. They were those scratchy plastic ones with the multi-coloured stripes, the ones you sit on at the beach and the sides of your bottom spill over the edges, so you end up with lines dug into your backside. I wondered if Evelyn had bought them for the occasion, as they looked new.

Environmental health had given her a few days to save anything significant before they cleared nearly everything out, she told me.

'It was impossible,' she shrugged. 'I didn't know what to do.'

In the end, she only managed to put a couple of items in a box and the rest was taken away. This had clearly upset her.

'They took it like it was all rubbish. I wish I had more time to sort things out properly.'

We sat in the chairs and I pulled out my notebook as Evelyn handed me some papers, which she fished out from the pile stacked in the corner.

The pathologist who had carried out Mairead's post-mortem examination stated she had fractured several ribs in a fall in the weeks leading up to her death, developing pneumonia as a result. She had osteoporosis and had seen the GP eight days before her death, complaining of pain in her sides following tripping and falling onto a metal plant stand. She'd refused to go to hospital. The report conceded that 'a fall of this nature from a standing height could fracture the ribs, particularly in an elderly lady susceptible by reason of osteoporosis'. There was no suspicion of foul play.

'A few days before she died, she had a dry cough and was breathless,' Evelyn explained, her voice starting to crack. 'So, she took to her bed.' Evelyn looked to the space where her sister's bed used to be.

'I couldn't decide whether or not to call the doctor, and then Mairead asked me to make her fish pie and peas, so I did that.'

When the meal was ready, Mairead got up and sat in the chair next to her bed, and she ate more than she'd eaten in weeks. Evelyn took that as a positive sign and decided not to call the doctor that night. In hindsight, she could see the meal was, as she put it, 'for the journey'. When she went to check on her sister later that evening, Mairead was cold in her bed.

Evelyn seemed to struggle to find the words to carry on with her story. After a moment, she looked at me and said very quietly, 'I lost her all at once.'

Clearly, Evelyn had found the suddenness of her sister's death an unbearable wrench.

At that time, I had no experience of losing a close family member. Then, this year, I lost my father and, though much time had passed since Mairead's death, her and Evelyn's story came back to me as I contemplated my own grief.

When my dad was dying, my mother and I were sitting by his bed when we saw his cheeks suddenly collapse inwards, with an audible *pop*. My mum gasped, recognizing it as a sign that he didn't have long left. My dad was in his bed at home, where he'd chosen to be, and we sat with him from 9am that morning until he passed away in the early hours of the next day. It felt like such a long, drawn-out process. I'd said what I wanted to say to him and all the important decisions had been made about his funeral and what he wanted to happen.

Death had never been a taboo subject in our family. 'Put me on a bonfire at the bottom of the garden,' he'd always joked, because he loved nothing better than a bonfire and hated the idea we'd waste any money on sausage rolls he'd never taste at a wake.

'I'll come back and haunt you if you do!' he'd warned.

After he passed, Mum, my sister and I all sat with him, waiting for the funeral director to come. It was the first time I'd ever been in the physical presence of a corpse, despite the countless dead bodies I'd pored over in the course of my work, on video and in photographs.

It wasn't macabre, though almost straight away Dad looked indefinably different. I've heard it said that this is the body's way of helping the bereaved process their loss by showing them that their loved one, as they knew them, has physically departed. I doubt that nature is that thoughtful. My dad turned dove grey, as his blood was no longer circulating, and his mouth relaxed open. Mum faffed around, smoothing down his hair, stroking his arm and gently grazing his forehead with her hand to close his eyes.

Dad hadn't eaten in weeks and once he'd been laid out in fresh pyjamas by the district nurses, he looked almost flat to the bed, like one of those little rubber skeletons they sell in joke shops. I don't know how long we sat there but I remember precisely how I felt when the funeral director arrived to take him away.

This is it. The last moment I'll ever spend with my dad.

The realization was a hard one to swallow.

Mum was feeling the finality too. She wanted to make sure they were not going to cover Dad's face or zip him unceremoniously into a body bag because she wanted him to be treated with care and dignity and nothing but respect.

'I'll treat him as though he's a member of my own family,' the funeral director promised.

We both thanked him and, though I didn't want to, I told my mum it was time now. We had to say goodbye.

When I kissed my dad's forehead, he felt smooth and cold. I'd told him that I loved him and how grateful I was to have had him as my father, which was really all I wanted to say.

Mum kissed him goodbye and we walked down the stairs together. It's very hard, knowing that's the last time you will see that person. But I was as ready as I could ever be and that helped a great deal.

Long before Dad died, I could see my new world without him taking shape. I stopped finding bits of his terrible DIY in my house. My garden became overgrown because he couldn't manage it the way he always did, without me even asking him to. Eventually, the only time I saw him was at Mum and Dad's house, not mine. And then, in the end, whenever I visited him, Dad was lying in his bed and another small piece of him was gone.

I thought about the John Irving novel, *A Prayer for Owen Meany*. There's a very moving section in it, about the death of a woman: 'You lose her in pieces over a long time – the way the mail stops coming, and her scent fades from the pillows and even from the clothes in her closet and drawers.'

Evelyn hadn't had the painful luxury that I'd had. She had lost her sister 'all at once', instead of in pieces over time. I wonder if losing someone more slowly, in increments, is easier than the shock Evelyn experienced at her finding her sister dead after eating a good meal, which she had felt sure was a positive step towards her recovery.

Overwhelmed, Evelyn couldn't decide who to phone or what to do. Just like she'd been unable to decide whether to call the doctor earlier that evening. I thought about the mountains of clutter. Every item in the house was a delayed decision of some sort, I thought.

'I sat with her for a bit. I didn't know whether she wanted to be buried or cremated. So I thought to cover her with her sheet and duvet while I figured out what to do.'

Evelyn couldn't figure out what to do, not that day or the day after. Then, after doing nothing for two days, shame kicked in. What would she say? Why had she not reported her sister's death straight away?

She bought the holy water and collected Mairead's pension, using the money to buy the magazines she would normally buy for her sister and leaving them on the bed beside her body. She also bought her gifts. New slippers, bags, knitting patterns and wool. She knew they were of no use to her but they were things she would have liked, she said. Evelyn also bought items for herself. 'Retail therapy,' she said ashamedly.

When Mairead's body started to smell, Evelyn piled the air fresheners on the pillow. After a week, she shut the bedroom door and didn't go back in.

It was such a terribly sad story. Though difficult for most people to contemplate, the situation Evelyn had found herself in was slowly making sense.

Evelyn said she wanted a cigarette and suggested we go out the back door. I was relieved. Not only was I desperate to breathe some fresh air, I would have been nervous that the place might go up like a tinderbox if Evelyn lit up inside.

'How did you and your sister come to live here together?' I asked, squishing myself into a patch of space in the small yard, which was packed with old electrical goods, broken bits of furniture and rusting garden tools.

Evelyn wheezed as she took a long drag on her cigarette. Then she cleared her throat and started to tell me about her background. I listened carefully, taking notes, as she recounted details of her childhood and upbringing, and the circumstances of her and her sister's move from Derry to the northwest of England.

Evelyn was the second youngest of nine children, raised in a very strict Catholic family. Mairead was 14 years her senior and Evelyn looked up to her like she was a second 'mini mum'. The family was extremely poor and their father hated waste of any kind. Every scrap of food had to be eaten, nothing useful ever thrown away and every item of clothing was mended and handed down from sibling to sibling.

Evelyn got a brand new Babykins doll for her tenth birthday and was so terrified that she'd eventually have to give it to her younger sister that she cut its hair and started hiding it at night.

'Mairead said I was always like a squirrel with its nuts.'

At 17, Evelyn fell pregnant. The father was a police officer she met when there was a theft at the dress shop where she worked. It was 1968, when The Troubles were brewing in Northern Ireland. Not only was the RUC officer a Protestant, which her father would have 'hit the roof' over, but he was also newly married. Evelyn tried to conceal the pregnancy under baggy clothes but her mother was too perceptive for it to remain secret for long. 'You cannot stay in this house,' she said.

Evelyn didn't know what to do but Mairead – a nursery-school teacher who was 'never one for the boys' – volunteered to bring her sister to England. She relished the chance of freedom from the family, Evelyn said. It was a fresh start and an exciting adventure for both of them.

The sisters arrived in the northwest when Evelyn was six months pregnant. Mairead found a job in a nursery and they moved into a rented terraced house. Evelyn was thrilled to bits when she got some part-time work as a seamstress and her employer brought round a sewing machine so she could work from home.

Best of all, the sisters had a bedroom each for the first time in their lives. They bought a record player – something their father would never have allowed – and set about buying bits of furniture and baby equipment, making their little house a home.

'It was the happiest time I can remember,' Evelyn said, smiling nostalgically.

She bought the Amen Corner record '(If Paradise Is) Half as Nice', which was at the top of the 'hit parade' at the time, and the sisters danced joyfully around the living room.

'I played it over and over again. I remember all the words. Every one.' She started singing some of the lyrics to '(If Paradise Is) Half As Nice' to me.

I remembered the song and joined in with the chorus.

'I'll never forget it,' she said, adding that after her baby was born – she had a son – she played it non-stop.

We'd started to pick our way back inside the bungalow now, Evelyn having finished her cigarette.

'I know all this needs sorting out,' she said, waving at the clutter. 'I do know that.'

This was the first time she'd acknowledged she had a problem, which was going to make my job a lot easier.

I asked her to talk me through some of her belongings while I continued to take notes, as picking over the haul of her life's memories was probably going to tell me more about her than any psychological test or questionnaire.

'Tell me about this,' I asked, randomly picking out a black porcelain cat that happened to be within reach (and looked like it wouldn't start an avalanche when I moved it).

The cat reminded her of one back in Northern Ireland that used to visit the family home, she said, giving a little smile at the memory. 'I absolutely loved that cat.'

'Can you imagine ever getting rid of it?'

'Oh, I don't know. If I threw this away I might forget about it; we called it Ringo because it had a white stripe round the end of its tail.'

A fold of material with cherry blossoms on it was earmarked for 'making something out of, one day'. It was stained and looked like it had festered there for a long while but Evelyn said it would be 'a terrible waste' to throw it away. Mind you, the two sewing machines she owned were buried somewhere in the chaos, so they would have to be found before she could get to work.

A broken plastic basket was a 'nice shape'. It was also very handy for storing birthday cards, which dated back several years. She talked me through some of them, obviously proud that she had plenty of friends and people who cared enough to send a card.

Evelyn told me her landlord had gone mad when he found out about the clutter (*as well as the dead body*, I thought, but didn't comment). He'd threatened to evict her if she didn't have a clear-out.

'I've been trying, I really have.' Evelyn had been moving bags and boxes from one room to another, constantly putting things in different piles but not, she admitted, actually getting rid of anything. A behaviour that psychologists describe as 'churning'.

She obviously felt overwhelmed, which was hardly surprising.

'I imagine it must be very difficult for you, to do it on your own.'

'Yes. Mairead helped me, but since she's been gone it's got worse and worse.'

Mairead used to put boundaries in place, like 'no magazines over two months old' or 'no food past its sell-by date'. Left to her own devices, Evelyn acknowledged her bedroom had become too overcrowded to use and she'd started sleeping on the armchair in the lounge.

I wanted to offer to pull on a pair of Marigolds, hire a skip (or three) and help Evelyn start the clear-out, but obviously I couldn't. It wasn't my place, though I did ask her permission to contact some specialist charities who could provide support.

She nodded in reluctant agreement.

Evelyn explained that she had friends at work she socialized with who hadn't been round for years.

'I suppose I've missed having people coming into the house,' she said. 'But there's not a lot of room for anyone to visit, is there?'

'No, there isn't.'

Evelyn told me she understood the way she lived was unusual and admitted she was ashamed of how bad the mess had become.

'What about your family?' I asked. 'Do they visit?'

She looked a bit taken aback by the question. I wondered if she'd become estranged from her family after leaving Ireland, but that wasn't the case.

'Some of them used to come but they haven't for a long time.'

I guessed her son would be in his forties now. 'What about your son? Does he visit you?"

'My son?'

She opened her mouth to speak but couldn't find any words for quite a few moments. My eyes flicked back over my notes. I was sure she had told me she had a son, but had I got that wrong? I found the relevant note and could see I hadn't. There it was in black and white.

Evelyn took a deep breath.

'Yes, I did have a son,' she said. 'I called him John.' When she said his name, she appeared to freeze.

I gave it a moment and then said, 'I remember you told me you played your Amen Corner record non-stop, after he was born.'

'Yes, I did. I played it for three days solid. But after three days, I couldn't stand to listen to the words any more. I broke the record into pieces.'

She looked around. 'It's in here somewhere. Maybe in

the wardrobe in my bedroom. I kept all the pieces. I'd like to find that record.' She added that she also wanted to find her old Babykins doll, the one she'd cut the hair off as a small girl in Ireland. The doll was also buried somewhere in the house.

'It isn't lost, though,' Evelyn said, as though reassuring herself.

'What happened to John?' I asked.

There was another pause, a longer one this time.

Evelyn swallowed hard. 'My son was stillborn.'

She said the words slowly and very quietly before explaining to me that the midwife whisked him away from her as soon as he was delivered, 'as they did in those days', believing they were saving bereaved mothers the trauma that a few precious moments together would cause.

'I did see him, though. I managed to get a little look at him as they took him away.'

The memory of that snatched look was all she had of him, she said.

Her mother told her that losing her child was 'probably for the best' and nobody besides Mairead ever mentioned John again. Her sister packed everything they had collected for him – cot, clothes, bottles, nappies and toys – into black sacks and got rid of the whole lot before Evelyn came home from hospital, thinking that would make it easier for her.

'One minute I was his mum and then he was gone, and it was as though he'd never been. I didn't know what I was going to do any more. I felt – I am still, empty.'

She had lost him – and her sense of identity – all at once, I realized.

She straightened herself up. 'It was a long time ago,' she said. 'I should have learned to live with it by now, shouldn't I?'

'No, I don't think so,' I answered.

The widely accepted view of grieving is encapsulated by the Five Stages of Grief model (described by Swiss-American psychiatrist Elisabeth Kübler-Ross in the 1969 classic book *On Death and Dying*) – shock/denial, anger, depression and bargaining, eventually arriving at acceptance. But despite its enduring popularity, science has not found any evidence, neither hide nor hair, of the existence of these stages. There is no road map for grief. It is not a time-limited or a linear process with steps to work through like levels on a PlayStation game. Like death itself, it's a very personal affair.

George Bonanno, professor of clinical psychology at Columbia University, interviewed hundreds of bereaved people and found that there is a wide range of grief patterns – anything from successful coping and mild grief reactions (feeling detached, having difficulty concentrating and being suddenly tearful, for example), to pernicious and lasting pain. The majority of us are surprisingly resilient when it comes to loss, though lasting grief is not uncommon, with between 10 and 15 per cent of people struggling with long-lasting sadness.

I didn't attend Evelyn's sentence hearing but an article in a local newspaper – under a lurid 'House of Horrors' headline – told me that she was given an 18-month suspended sentence and was ordered to pay back the stolen pension money. She wasn't ordered to take part in any psychiatric treatment. 'Hoarding disorder' wasn't yet a thing (it didn't appear in the *Big Book of Human Suffering* until 2013). And perhaps the judge realized, as I did, that she wasn't suffering from 'depression' but from grief. Catastrophic, unabating grief. In my report, I'd said she needed gentle assistance to clear her home, combined with help to make sense of why she had felt the need to hold on to so many pieces of her life.

Feeling like an empty room can be what inspires us to fill one. We all take comfort from material 'stuff', to some extent. 'More than mere tools, luxuries or junk, our possessions become extensions of the self,' says Christian Jarrett, writing on 'the psychology of stuff and things'. 'We use them to signal to ourselves, and others, who we want to be and where we want to belong. And long after we're gone, they become our legacy. Some might even say our essence lives on in what once we made or owned.'

Stuff reminds us of our childhood, of happy times in our lives and of people we love who are absent or deceased. But trend forecaster James Wallman warns that, increasingly, we have more things than we could ever need and the focus on possessions rather than experience only serves to make us more stressed. 'Overwhelmed, and suffocating from stuff, we are suffering from an anxiety that I call "Stuffocation",' he writes.

Evelyn was stuffocated. In her case, hoarding had become her way of coping with loss. So deep was the tear in her sense of self when she had lost her son, she could not let go of anything. A decades-old broken record. Her sister's corpse.

Mairead's body was cremated and Evelyn kept her ashes in a silver urn, while she decided what to do with them.

CHAPTER SEVEN

PORK AND PREJUDICE

'Where are all the residents?' I asked.

It was late on Monday morning and the drug-rehabilitation project felt like a ghost ship.

'They haven't got up yet,' the flushed-cheeked manager told me. 'We suspect there was some drug-taking at the weekend.'

Looking decidedly peeved, he began describing how four residents were up all night dancing, 'even when we turned the music off'. Another man had spent the whole night huddled up in a corner in a 'state of paranoia' and someone else had become 'far too affectionate, trying to hug everyone in sight'.

As he expelled a sigh of displeasure from deep within his barrel-like chest, I found myself suppressing a wry smile. Of course those residents were in bed. They'd have to pay back the biological bank this morning. Anyone dancing to nothing more than the beat of a dripping tap all night long had probably taken some kind of stimulant drug – 'ecstasy' (MDMA) being my best guess. For the manager to say he 'suspected' them of spending the weekend in an altered state but not to have initiated any drug testing seemed either endearingly generous or worryingly naïve. I didn't want to jump to the latter conclusion because, despite his rather statesman-like physique, Robert – 'but call me Bobby, everyone else here does' – was young for a manager. He was still clinging onto his twenties, I imagined.

'What about the others?' I asked, looking around hopefully.

Bobby raised half of his bushy black monobrow. 'Others? There are no other residents.'

So the 'everyone else here' amounted to just six residents, a deputy manager and a handful of support workers, plus a psychiatrist who visited every other Thursday.

'We did have 13 residents to start with,' Bobby explained, 'but we have a policy of asking the men to leave if they're found using non-prescription drugs.'

He delivered this line deadpan and with no hint of irony. How on earth did that policy translate to a drug-rehab unit? Now things were making more sense, though. This manager wasn't going as far as to drug-screen his last remaining residents as he'd be doing himself out of a job!

The rehab unit was in a large, Regency-style house that appeared quite grand from the long winding track leading up to it. Set in acres of rolling countryside in a remote part of Yorkshire, it could have provided the backdrop for a period drama. Sadly for its neighbours, such an honour had never been bestowed upon it. Formerly a charity-run forensic step-down project, it had been hastily repurposed after locals discovered it housed a sprinkling of former sex offenders. They banded together in protest. 'Nonces out!' read the placards. 'We don't want sex offenders in our village!' It is an understandable concern, although somebody should have told them that, in all likelihood, they already *had* sex offenders in their village, just not ones who had been discovered, served time in prison and were now being carefully supervised in one large house.

Regardless of the lack of logic in the NIMBY-brigade's argument, the unwanted men were shipped out, only for the 15-bed house, adjoining cottage and outhouses to be turned – very recently – into a (somewhat) more acceptable-sounding 'substance misuse recovery site'. I'd love to have been a fly on the wall at the parish-council meeting when that news came up in 'any other business'.

The grand house still offered a home for male ex-offenders (just not the least welcome kind). The new facility was a place where those with 'dual diagnosis' – problem drug use and mental-health problems – would be able to rehabilitate back into society via a programme of therapies, on-site activity and support to access nearby education and employment. A thoroughly laudable mission, but financial pressure to fill the beds meant that residents had arrived fresh from prisons and secure hospitals almost before the newly appointed staff – who between them had no direct experience in addiction services – had drawn breath. Not surprisingly, they were desperately unprepared and in need of direction and support.

I'd been hired for six weeks in spring 2010 to help Bobby come up with a viable strategy to get the place operational as an actual rehabilitation unit, rather than just a two-star hotel. Six weeks wasn't nearly long enough but it was all his budget could stretch to.

In that short period, I'd need to work out what the project could offer in terms of therapy, write up the associated policies and paperwork, put the basics of a therapeutic programme in place and decide how to spend what was left in the charity's dusty coffers. It was a process I had been through several times before in hospitals I'd worked in but, even so, faced with the raw materials I had to work with, I was feeling I may have bitten off more than I could chew.

'You can use this as your base,' Bobby said, opening a door to a huge main office and pointing out a rosewood desk in the far corner. 'I'll go and find the staff. Hopefully they can get the residents out of their beds. Feel free to take a look around. That's the TV lounge, directly opposite.'

I watched him climb a wide, creaking staircase, his heavy footsteps echoing around the wooden-floored reception area. The place was eerily quiet and I almost felt I should be tiptoeing as I crossed the hallway and pushed open the heavy double doors of the TV lounge.

I stopped in my tracks, blinking at the migraine-inducing floral wallpaper, clashing borders and collection of stuffed small animals displayed on a dark mahogany dresser. A dead-eyed weasel was baring its teeth at me. *Just what you'd need when you're on a drugs comedown*, I thought. Feeling increasingly like a doomed guest in a B-movie horror, I took in the rest of the faded décor. Washed-out mustard-coloured pelmets capped long, swirly-patterned curtains and several plaid-checked sofas were dotted around, each one sagging in the middle, crushed by time and apathy.

Across the back of the room, in front of an empty fireplace, stood a full-size pool table. *Surely nobody wants to hear the clonk of balls being potted when they're watching telly*, I thought.

All the residents had an extensive substance-misuse history, a list of drug-related convictions to their names and were at high risk of falling back into familiar ways. This was their last-chance saloon, but if they stayed the course and successfully completed up to two years of rehabilitation they might break the cycle of relapse and reoffending. Cornily, 'Hotel California' started playing in my head. These guests didn't have the luxury of being able to check out any time they liked, but would they ever truly leave?

Just at that moment, a gust of wind roared from the bowels of the fireplace, causing one of the pool balls to plop noisily into the nearest pocket. I jumped like a flea on a trampoline.

I was invited to sit in on the afternoon's Substance Awareness Group, which two of the support workers were running and all the men were due to attend. Bobby explained it was an educational package, downloaded from the internet and focusing on the different types of street drugs and their potential effects. The popularity of 'awareness' programmes, covering everything from problematic pornography use, domestic abuse and the ubiquitous 'mental-health awareness', took off in the 1990s and has never abated. Raising consciousness and understanding of issues is, of course, a good and necessary thing. But too many services offer up these groups as though they provide a comprehensive answer to people's problems, which isn't how it works. As the vast majority of us know, having an *awareness* of something doesn't automatically lead to a willingness or ability to *do* anything about it. My brain, for instance, is fully aware that eating a tube of Pringles for breakfast is not the most nutritious start to the day, but the pleasure of doing so far outweighs my intellectual understanding when faced with a cupboard of temptation and a decision to make.

Still, I needed to see for myself what was being provided before I made any judgements. The staff had clearly been struggling to fill the hours. Although something told me that this group of residents was already highly educated in the subject on offer, as Bobby had said, 'We've got to deliver *something*.'

I went into the session with an open mind. The support workers – a youngish blonde woman and a freckle-faced man in his late thirties – were setting themselves up with a flip-chart at one end of a high-ceilinged room where the raised ornate mouldings in the plaster were covered in paint that looked several decades thick. The staff looked self-conscious but both were friendly enough towards me, saying hello and inviting me to sit down.

'This is Kerry Daynes, everyone,' said the woman. 'She's a psychologist and she's here to help us improve the unit.'

The residents barely looked up. I counted six of them. At least the staff had managed to shoehorn them all out of bed, though only just, by the looks of it. The men were sprawled on a series of hard wingback chairs. Without exception, they looked worn down, lethargic and completely disengaged.

What I wasn't prepared for was how I felt the moment I was introduced. An unwelcome feeling was creeping through me, one I didn't immediately recognize or comprehend, and that took me completely by surprise. I was unnerved, I realized. It was something I hadn't anticipated and I tried to work out why I felt the way I did. It wasn't the demeanour of the men that triggered my response to them. I'm used to walking into a room full of strangers and I'm often the one who has to stand at the front and deliver the training to an audience that isn't exactly thrilled to be there. The fact that the residents had a large collection of drug convictions and mental-health diagnoses between them didn't come into the equation either. I'd been working with ex-offenders with mental-health problems for the best part of 15 years – many of whom had committed vastly more hair-raising crimes than these guys.

No. Loath as I am to admit it, what unsettled me was that all the residents were Black and all the staff were white. And the obvious and unexpected division is what had set off an alarm bell I didn't expect to hear.

That's racist, I thought. *But I'm not a racist!*

Isn't protesting against the accusation of racism often the first line of defence when a person is called out on it, as though the accusation of it is somehow worse than the act itself?

It was not an easy conversation to have, even in the privacy of my own thoughts. *If there wasn't a problem here, why would you feel unnerved by a group of men with different colour skin?*

Black men and boys are scandalously overrepresented in prisons, and Black people are four times more likely to be sectioned and put in locked mental-health services than their white counterparts. I'd worked with many BAME clients over the years, yet here I was, thrown off kilter by this all-Black group.

John Dovidio, a professor of psychology and public health at Yale University, argues that racism has (for the most part) become far more subtle since the civil rights movement of the 1950s and 60s. 'Instead of feelings of hatred,' he says, contemporary prejudice is 'more like feelings of avoidance and discomfort'.

Even if you consider yourself an ally of people of colour, cognizant of the multitude of ways that our systems discriminate against BAME communities, you may still be holding 'unconscious bias'. That is to say, the stereotypical attitudes and beliefs about certain groups of people that filter through our culture so insidiously that we are not even fully aware we have them. The consideration for psychologists is not *whether* we hold biases of any kind but the extent to which we are prepared to notice them and then (bearing in mind the problem with 'awareness' groups) act to prevent them having a negative impact on our work.

I was dismayed at how deftly my little share of racial bias had popped up despite all my declared values and beliefs. Negative associations had managed to infiltrate my psyche. I wondered what lurked just out of reach in the minds of the rest of the exclusively white staff group. More to the point, how might the glaring split, not just in the racial make-up of residents and staff but in the power that only one of those groups held, impact on the unit?

Nevertheless, one of the best ways to mitigate against unconscious bias is simply to meet with and interact with people as individuals, and here was my opportunity.

'What are the different street names for cannabis?' the blonde woman was asking.

The men had lolled even further back in their seats, none making the slightest effort to even pretend to be interested.

'Ganja,' offered a bald-headed man after a pained pause. That was the sole contribution.

The young woman started listing all the different names for cannabis on the flip-chart, copying diligently from a list. Dope. Mary Jane. Blow. Skunk. The last caught the attention of one resident, who pinged his eyes open to comment, 'That's the good stuff!'

Another retorted, 'I could have used some of that last night.'

'With your paranoia?' the first man replied. 'Man, you need something ultra mellow. Kush. Or Northern Lights.'

A couple of the others nodded sagely. This was a perfect opportunity to segue into the expectations and reality of cannabis use but neither member of staff used it to their advantage. Instead, they ploughed on, taking it in turns to read from the dry notes in their neatly bound course packs. It was a tough crowd, the pupils evidently knowing more than the teachers.

I sat in contemplative silence, watching the canyon between the staff and the residents grow wider.

'Let me hand over to Kerry,' said the freckled man, looking relieved. 'As we said, she is here to help make this a better drug-rehab centre.'

Bracing myself, I sat bolt upright in my chair. 'I appreciate you all being here, as I can see you are dealing with the effects of what was clearly a heavy weekend.'

The men looked so bored they could barely muster one look of acknowledgement between them.

'But I'm really interested in your opinions and ideas for what this place could offer. What would be a help in getting you closer to where you want to be in life?'

The silence was as thick as the paint on the ceiling.

After ten long minutes of getting precisely nowhere, I changed tack. There was nothing to be gained from pussy-footing around and so I braced myself again and told it how it was. 'The first thing that hit me when I walked into this room today is that you are all Black and all of the staff I've met here are white.'

The two members of staff looked like they'd just been tasered, while the bald man – Danjuma – let out a long, high-pitched 'Hooooo!' His smile told me he appreciated me pointing so boldly at the elephant in the room, but it was another man, Isaaq, who picked up the baton.

'It's standard, innit? Everywhere I go. If you want to know who's in charge, it's the white man.'

Suddenly the men were no longer dozing and all eyes were

firmly focused on me. I nodded at Isaaq.

'I'd like to hear what all of you think about it,' I said. 'Is it something that you notice day to day?'

'It's not just this place that's all white,' another man said.

He explained that the surrounding villages were filled exclusively with white faces. It meant that whenever the men went out to use the local facilities they suffered a double whammy of suspicion because not only did they stand out for being Black, everyone in the local area knew where they came from.

'Might as well have "junkie" stamped on our faces,' piped up the quietest resident in the room.

'Nah, you don't need to spell it out, man,' Isaaq said. 'That's the whole point. You can see women clutching their handbags closer when you get near. They look the other way, cross the road. They think I'm some kind of savage. It's all they see. No need for a stamp. Your skin is your label. Simple as.'

The men were becoming more animated, all six giving something to the conversation. I learned that the hairdressers in the village claimed not to know how to cut Black hair, the toiletries in the unit were not suitable for the men's skin, there was nowhere to buy the oil they needed for their beards and the food served was too bland for their palates.

I'd never considered going to a hairdressers and being told they didn't know what to do with my hair, or not being able to easily buy the right shampoo. And that's despite the fact I belong in the minority group of people with the melanocortin 1 receptor (MC1R), meaning I'm one of the less than 2 per cent of the global population who are redheads.

For want of a good barber, most of the men in the room had longer hair, piled high on their heads or worn as afros. Statistically speaking, they had hair that was infinitely more common than mine but the billions of others in the world with Black hair had not found themselves planted in the wilds of Yorkshire.

'Sometimes it can make you feel like you have less right just to be in a place,' the youngest-looking man told me.

The men started having a deeper conversation, among themselves.

'At one school I went to, I was the only Black kid in the class,' the young man continued. 'You know what I did? I got a scrubbing brush and tried to scrub the blackness off my skin.'

'Whaaat! Who d'you think you are!' Danjuma laughed, his bald head shining under the wall lights. 'Michael Jackson?'

Isaaq – who had the biggest crown of natural curls of the lot, as well as the most charismatic smile – thought this was funny. He playfully pushed the shoulder of the young man, while Danjuma pointed his finger at his housemates. 'Look at you lot sitting there with your afros, we've got the whole Jackson 5!'

It was well-meaning banter, designed to soothe a painful admission, but the two staff looked startled. They were exchanging worried looks about where the conversation was going to take us and perhaps whether we should even be having it.

'Why did you scrub yourself?' Isaaq frowned. 'Were you ashamed, man? Ashamed of being Black?'

'No, but as a kid it was like Muhammad Ali said, you know what I mean?' Some of the men started to nod knowingly but he elaborated nonetheless. 'It made me think about being Black and why everything we were told about it was bad. You get a black mark against your name. The black cat was bad luck. You fall into a black mood. And I didn't want to be a black sheep or be the odd one out.'

'Don't hate yourself, brother,' Danjuma said, kindly. 'There's enough to go round,' he added.

The group fell back into a reflective stillness.

'So, what happened here over the weekend?' I ventured.

Danjuma, who had been one of the all-night dancers, folded his arms and said nothing. Again it was Isaaq who spoke up first.

'That was bad gear,' he said, shaking his head. Isaaq had evidently been the one who was curled up in a terrified ball all night.

'Bad, bad gear. That's what happened. Pills take me to a bad place.'

'You know they take you to a bad place,' I replied, 'so it sounds like things got out of hand.'

He waved his hand around the room. 'Yeah, but there's nothing else to do here. I just wanted to have a break for a few hours, you know?'

Cue more nodding heads.

'What would you like to be doing while you are here?' I asked.

Isaaq said they didn't need lectures on cannabis or classes informing them of the different ways that people take heroin. 'We *know* that,' he said slowly, pointing to the left side of his face. The eye socket was large and the lid closed, his eyeball missing, the result of an untreated infection caused by injecting into it with a dirty needle.

'Talking about drugs just makes me crave some,' said the youngest man.

'So, we know what isn't helpful, what *would* be helpful?' I prompted.

Isaaq shook his head.

'Let me put it another way, when you were feeling your most positive about coming here, what were you hoping for?'

It was Danjuma who eventually answered. 'Just to be somewhere that believes I can do better.'

The next morning, I sat in my cold corner of the office sketching out a treatment model I hoped was ambitious enough to be effective yet simple enough to be practical.

Sitting in a huge box on my desk, I had a groupwork programme I'd made earlier, in true *Blue Peter* style, in my former life as a secure-hospital psychologist. It addressed the links between substance use and offending and, with some careful reworking, it would make the ideal backbone to therapy at the project, targeting as it did the specific psychological and social skills the men needed to stop them spiralling into relapse. The programme would need to be backed up with individually tailored one-to-one therapy and support because otherwise we would simply be jumping from one 'one-size-fits-all' intervention to another, albeit a more sophisticated, one. It was crucial that we hired someone with the multitude of talents needed to deliver the programme well.

I'd already agreed with Bobby that a nine-to-five post for an activities coordinator needed to be created. This person would not only oversee my vision for a house that had appealing pursuits at its core, but he or she would make links in the community and explore whatever opportunities existed in the neighbouring towns. The money left in the charity's purse wouldn't stretch to hiring a psychologist but we could, however, afford a specialist drugs counsellor. And I knew just the multi-skilled professional for the job, one who just happened to come with an advantageous, hairy sidekick.

Gavin was an experienced police officer and dog handler who had quit South Yorkshire Police several years earlier to retrain as an independent drug counsellor and psychotherapist. He'd made the switch after his best friend and co-worker, a sniffer dog called Dougie, found a stash of heroin in the cellar of a middle-class family alongside the emaciated body of a teenage girl. She was just 15 – the same age as Gavin's daughter at the time – and she'd been trafficked from Romania and forced to act as a drugs mule.

Gavin was delighted to apply for the role at the project and would even show the staff how to conduct room searches, ticking off one item on my list of training needs. Being able to bring Dougie to work was his ideal set-up. His experience of dog handling had stemmed from his farming background in Yorkshire, where he'd trained gundogs and working sheepdogs.

'He's absolutely ideal,' I said to the deputy manager, Rory, who had only been in post himself for a couple of months.

'If you say so,' he said, warily.

'I do,' I smiled, pointing out how difficult it was to recruit *anyone* in such a rural location. 'He couldn't be more perfect for the job. Well, not unless he was Black.'

Rory looked at me in a way I couldn't fathom. If it was disapproval, it seemed woefully misplaced, given that by now I'd spoken to him and Bobby about the racial disparity and how we needed to address it, not least by attracting some good BAME staff. 'Get over yourself,' I felt like saying.

It was day ten – a Friday – when I introduced our two new recruits to the unit.

With his pink complexion, lack of hair, squat build and disproportionately muscled arms, Gavin had always reminded me of a Disney crab. I don't mean that unkindly – he was a very knowledgeable, sensitive and approachable crab, and a great crustacean to have on your side. Dougie, meanwhile, was a beautiful brown and white beagle who had two settings – frantic activity or snoring (and farting) loudly. When he found drugs he would stop and stare, like a Pompeii pet frozen in time by the erupting Mount Vesuvius. His full title was, inevitably, Dougie the Druggie Dog.

Next week will be interesting, I thought, imagining Dougie playing musical statues in at least one resident's room, because somebody had to be responsible for bringing drugs into the facility. Room searches and sniffer dogs are not the most conducive to creating an atmosphere of unity between staff and residents, but if we were ever going to disperse the heavy cloud of hopelessness that hung over the project and encourage residents to lead the charge in their own recovery, we would need to tackle the supply of drugs to the place. At least the policy of issuing an eviction notice to anyone found using illicit substances had been ripped up and replaced with something more reasonable, that didn't see residents out on their ear. Instead, the emphasis would be on the management of any short-term risks and consideration of the essential question of 'Why lapse now?'

I was surprised to learn that Isaaq had become the prime suspect in the search for a magic Skittles peddler. Rory explained to me and Gavin that he had been involved in drug-dealing from a young age. Not only that, staff members had reported that Isaaq had seemed 'off-hand' with them over the past few weeks.

'We've stopped all residents going on unescorted leave outside,' Rory said. 'Hopefully that will disrupt the supply chain.'

The men at the project loved Dougie, his soulful brown eyes winning over even the most outwardly indifferent among them. Despite his flatulence and olfactory superpowers, every resident seemed chuffed to have a dog around the place.

At the end of the day, with the weekend firmly in my sights, Bobby let me out of the panelled front door and walked with me towards my car. Gavin and Danjuma were outside, chatting on a bench on the lawn while throwing a saliva-sodden tennis ball for an over-excited Dougie. Waving, they threw the ball over to us but Dougie was already a few feet ahead of it, running to say hello, and he swiftly doubled back to catch it before dropping it at my feet.

As I bent to collect the ball, Gavin got up off the bench and hinged his muscle-bound arms above his head, ready for a catch.

'Are you ready, Dougie?' I said, waving the ball in the air. But Dougie had lost interest in the game, suddenly running over to the car parked next to mine on the driveway. Now he was standing as still as stone, staring intently at the back of it. There was not a flicker of movement in his body as his eyes were fixed, unmoving, on his prize.

Danjuma let out the same amused, falsetto whoop that he had in the Substance Awareness Group.

Twenty minutes later, Bobby and I were back in the office. The deputy manager, Rory, had been hauled in too, only to be told he was out on his ear – suspended with immediate effect. He cleared his desk in silence, barely having the good grace to look embarrassed. There was no point in arguing or denying it because Dougie had caught him red-handed. For there on Bobby's desk, for all to see, was a freezer bag full of ecstasy tablets and paper wrappers containing white powder. All of which had been retrieved from a lunchbox in the boot of Rory's Volkswagen Golf.

The following Monday, it felt like a tension had been massaged out of the place. Gavin and I had spent a productive morning training support workers in the use of the Recovery Star, a tool for promoting and measuring change. The 'star' contains ten aspects of people's lives, one being 'addictive behaviour', with others including 'identity and self-esteem', 'work', 'relationships', 'trust and hope' and so on. Residents are asked to set their personal goals within each aspect of the star and, as time goes on, measure how far they are progressing. Ideally, residents and their key worker should work together to identify what a life of meaning and purpose looks like to them and what support they need to help get them there. The quality of the conversations that take place around the different areas are infinitely more vital than the targets that are set or how far or how fast a person can plot their progress and so, like any tool, the usefulness of the Recovery Star depends on who is using it, and how.

I'd seen little evidence of relationships between staff and residents that could be described as based on listening, trust and empathy. Communication was functional: 'It's your day for laundry, have you got washing powder?' and 'I need to post a letter, can you sign me out?' If this place was going to turn a corner, that needed to change – and fast. So I crossed my fingers that Gavin and I had sown the first seeds of a new, therapeutic dialogue.

By lunchtime, I was eating strawberry Angel Delight (a personal favourite, but I had to agree with the men that the menu lacked a certain pizzazz) when Isaaq came dashing into the dining room, midriff bared as he clutched something to him, hidden in the makeshift hammock of his sweater.

'I found it on the side of the road,' he puffed.

'What is it?' I asked nervously. It was pink, wet and wrinkly, but that's where the similarity with my dessert ended. Whatever it was, this thing was alive and wriggling.

Isaaq angled his body so I could see the creature's head. It was a newborn piglet, so newborn, in fact, it still had its umbilical cord attached. The sight of it finally made me put down my spoon.

'There's an abattoir not far from here,' Gavin chipped in. 'Sometimes pregnant sows give birth in the truck on the way to be slaughtered. The little things fall out of the slats at the side and land on the road. Lucky you found this one, Isaaq.'

'What are we going to do with him?' Isaaq asked.

It transpired that I was the only member of staff whose car insurance allowed me to ferry residents around. Isaaq swiftly wrapped the piglet in a blanket, popped it in a sports bag and I drove as quickly as possible to the nearest vet. A support worker came with us, as I was only a contractor, rather than an official staff member. She navigated from the back seat as Isaaq apologized to our precious cargo for the sharp bends.

When we entered the waiting room at the vets, we joined a middle-aged man with a wiry terrier straining at the leash, a woman with a child, a young couple with what could have been a guinea pig, or possibly a sick hairpiece, and a pensioner with a covered basket at her feet. They all checked us out, either with a 'discreet' side eye or a more brazen once-over, like we were suspects in an identity parade.

Isaaq went to take the seat next to the pensioner, who

shifted slightly in her seat, moving the plastic basket at her feet by just an inch. Isaaq gave her a big smile.

'Don't worry, I'm harmless,' he said.

She gave the thinnest of smiles in return.

'It's a piglet,' he continued, gesturing towards the holdall (not that she'd asked). Isaaq pulled the blanket back to give the creature some air. The pensioner clearly didn't know what to say but she craned her neck to take a look. To be absolutely fair, despite his lightbulb smile, Isaaq looked like he'd had a tough paper round and his appearance naturally begged some questions.

A man with a missing eye and a literal pig-in-blanket in a sports bag was an unusual sight, even in these rural parts. Especially in these rural parts.

The woman looked at me as I tucked my car keys into my suit pocket. Then she glanced at my colleague, a sensibly-shod 40-something with grey-flecked hair. She was obviously trying, and failing, to put a context to this peculiar picture.

'My cat has an overactive thyroid,' she said. 'What's wrong with your pig?'

'I've no eye-dear!' replied Isaaq, pointing to his face.

The receptionist interjected. 'Excuse me, does your pet have a name?' she trilled, her voice cutting straight across the room.

She was looking between me and the support worker, even though Isaac was the one who was holding the piglet.

'PC Rasher,' Isaaq boomed back.

She arched an immaculately pencilled eyebrow. 'Can you spell that?'

We left the vet with considerably less money in the petty-cash tin and what felt like a rapid diploma in pig husbandry. Before sending us on our way with some replacement powdered milks and an eye-dropper, the vet had explained how PC Rasher would at first need to be hand-fed in small quantities, 15 times in every 24-hour period. Isaaq was more than happy to assume the role of chief caregiver, drawing up a feeding and cleaning roster and asking the other residents to pitch in. Only one man refused, declaring, 'I ain't touchin' no pig!' Unconscious bias of a different kind, I mused, because PC Rasher was nothing like the stereotype of a smelly, greedy and mud-splattered farm animal. Odourless and soft-skinned, *she* (as it turned out) was really quite adorable.

On the subject of 'negative associations', after some discussion, it was agreed that it might be wise to drop PC from the pig's name.

'It stands for Politically Correct, not Police Constable,' laughed Isaaq.

'Pull the other one,' I said.

The vet had told us such a tiny piglet wasn't able to regulate her body temperature and it could prove fatal if Rasher wasn't kept warm. Isaaq fashioned a bed out of a sturdy cardboard box and filled it with blankets and a hot-water bottle, and staff and residents pitched in to help clear the clutter from a spare room in the warmest part of the house, turning it into a temporary piglet nursery.

That first night, when I got back to the comfort of my own home, I found myself preoccupied, willing the pig not to die.

Isaaq was already looking at her in the same way that Gavin looked at Dougie and it had been fantastic to see everyone pulling together to help care for our new resident.

It was a relief to get to work the next morning and find Rasher not just alive but looking very much at home and in rude health. Isaaq, on the other hand, looked as shell-shocked and shattered as any new parent, having volunteered himself to oversee the first nightshift.

'I've barely slept a wink,' he said, wiping his brow with the back of his hand.

We learned that Rasher had a piercing screech, which Isaaq could hear from 50 paces. To be honest, I think most of the village could hear it but Isaaq was always first on hand, dashing to his charge's aid like a clucking mother hen.

I spent a lot of my time in the office that week, working through the core treatment programme with Gavin and putting together a training course for staff so that they could help facilitate it. But we needed to crawl before we could walk and so we put together a basic counselling-skills curriculum too. Every few hours, I wandered along to check on Rasher. At least that was the plan, because something else had started to take my attention.

'See this?' It was the youngest resident, the one who'd shared with the group how he tried to scrub his skin white. He was taking his turn with the feeding. 'Reminds me of when I used to feed my son, when he was being weaned. Man, I miss him so much.'

'I didn't know you had a baby,' the freckled member of staff asked. 'How long is it since you saw him?'

'Way too long. When I was off my head on drugs I was too ashamed of myself, you know? I didn't want myself around him.'

The men had set up chairs in Rasher's makeshift pen. It had fast become the hub of the project, support workers and residents dipping in and out with warmed milk, clean blankets and hay for her to root in. And in among the feeds and the cleaning, something happened, completely organically. They all started talking, about anything and everything. Even Bobby, and the man who'd refused to get his hands dirty, had turned up for a natter.

During one of my visits, I heard Isaaq mention how he'd felt when he'd arrived back in the UK after spending time in Somalia, his mother's homeland.

'I was like this little runt,' he said, stroking the sleeping pig on his lap. 'In a strange place with no family. When she fell out of the truck she must have been thinking, man, what the fuck is happening now?' He let out one of his raucous laughs.

I'd had a look at all the residents' notes and knew that Isaaq had been born in England, the youngest of four siblings. Their father left them when Isaaq was three, at which point their mother went back to Somalia with her four children. When ten-year-old Isaaq returned to the UK alone he was placed in foster care in Bristol.

'They put me with a good family,' I heard him telling the group. 'But I didn't belong there.'

Due to a lack of more culturally appropriate carers, he'd been placed with a white family. On the day that he arrived, he overheard his foster-father comment, 'The little lad's as black as the ace of spades,' a saying he'd never heard before and didn't understand. As a 'term of endearment', he called Isaaq his little pirate – a reference to the hijacking of foreign vessels off the coast of Somalia that was making international headlines at the time.

'It wasn't cool,' Isaaq told me. 'The kids at school picked up on it. They called me a Somalian pirate. I'd arrived on a boat but I was no pirate. Even the Black kids called me that.'

These days, his foster-father's language would be considered shockingly ignorant. But in late 1980s Britain it was commonplace enough to pass by unnoticed and unchallenged. 'No malice was intended,' Isaaq pointed out. Though regardless of intention, pain had been inflicted nonetheless.

'What happened to your real family, brother?' asked Danjuma. The blonde support worker nodded eagerly but Isaaq just waved his arm around dismissively.

'Somalia was a dangerous place,' he said.

Turning his attention back to Rasher, who was dribbling in her sleep, he added, 'You've got it easy, you know that? You've landed on your trotters, you lucky girl!'

Rasher certainly was a fortunate pig, in more ways than one. I'd heard that in Korea they believe that pigs signify good fortune and, if one appears in your dream, you will have great luck. Since her unexpected arrival at the project, a sense of cooperation had started to emerge, more potent than could ever be created by contrived team-building exercises. Having a mutual interest and purpose, and feeling part of a successful endeavour, was benefiting all. A stroke of incredible luck.

However, it was time to create more shared experiences beyond the pigsty, and so I called a meeting with residents and staff alike to come up with ideas.

'We have an activities coordinator starting in a month, so he is going to need some activities to coordinate. What skills and interests do you have that you could share with the rest of us? Could you put on a class, run a course?'

I'm the first to say, 'If you don't ask you don't get', and the policy started to pay off straight away. Every single resident and member of staff had something to offer, one or two taking us all by surprise.

Danjuma, for instance, had been trained by the Samaritans as a 'listener' when he was in prison, providing a confidential ear for fellow inmates who were finding it difficult to cope. So he was immediately recruited to partner with Gavin and help teach our basic counselling course to the staff and any residents who also wanted to join. Another man was a fan of spoken-word poetry, so he agreed to take the minutes of the weekly community meeting, converting them into a performance at the next meeting.

One of the female support workers – a particularly attractive young woman – had qualifications in yoga and meditation and offered to run weekly classes. Funnily enough, her groups were always full, with staff and residents vying for floor space whenever she was on shift. Another support worker had previously worked in construction and he and a couple of the men started building a pig pen in one of the outhouses. Those who knew a thing or two about gardening began creating a plan for the outdoor space, including a sty and run. It couldn't be built soon enough – after two weeks, Rasher was piling on weight, drinking noisily from a tin pan and rapidly outgrowing her cardboard sleeping quarters.

For his part, Gavin had started sharing his dog-training skills with Isaaq and Danjuma, teaching Rasher to sit. I kid you not. The pig was as obedient as they come, plonking her rapidly expanding backside down on her curly tail on command. If only there was a porcine version of Crufts, she'd have been top of her category!

The days were filling up and, though there was a mountain of work still to do, at least some kind of structure was bedding in.

'Can we get some ostriches?' the men asked me one day, when Rasher was under the pool table in the television room, snorting appreciatively.

'No, we can't! We're still learning about pigs! You need to start smaller. Why not ask Bobby for a few chickens?'

It was great to see them so enthusiastic, but don't be misled. While connections were forming and commonalities were revealed, the place hadn't suddenly transformed into a utopia. The staff and residents weren't exactly sitting around a campfire every nightfall singing 'Kumbaya'.

'How much money d'you reckon you could make from the disposal of dead bodies?' I overheard someone say one evening. The men were eating dinner, having watched *Hannibal*, the sequel to *Silence of the Lambs*, a few nights earlier.

'Why? What you thinking?' asked Danjuma.

'Rasher. She could eat people. I met people in prison that would pay good money for that shit...'

'Oi, I heard that. You better not be thinking of getting that pig involved in crime!' I shouted, reaching for the salt.

As my six weeks at the project counted down, Isaaq had continued sharing bits of his story, and I looked forward to the moments I could spend time with him and learn more.

I discovered that when Isaaq's dad walked out on the family, his mother took him and his three older brothers to live with her relatives back in Burao, Somalia. All his brothers had been born in Somalia, while Isaaq had come into the world in the back bedroom of the family's rented house in Birmingham, in 1978.

There was a rich historical backdrop to their situation, which I read up on. Britain, France and Italy had established colonies in the Horn of Africa in the 1800s and Somali seamen working on British ships started to settle in UK port cities. When merchant-navy jobs began to dry up in the 1960s, Somali families moved from the ports to industrial cities like Birmingham and Manchester. Meanwhile, the British and Italian colonies of Somaliland and Somalia had become fully independent, merging to form the United Republic of Somalia. President Mohamed Siad Barre held dictatorial rule over the country, after staging a coup in the wake of the assassination of former president Abdi Rashid Ali Shermarke in 1969. Isaaq told me that was the reason his parents had moved their family to the UK, joining relatives who had previously settled in Birmingham.

By the 1980s, the president faced huge opposition after filling governmental positions with members of his own clan while excluding members of other clans, including the one to which Isaaq and his family belonged. In 1981, as three-year-old Isaaq and his family were settling into Burao, clan-based guerrillas were plotting to overthrow the president.

As Isaaq grew from a toddler to a young boy, opposition escalated. Somalis started to flee the unrest, many arriving in British coastal cities as refugees. Isaaq, his mother and siblings stayed put but, by 1987, a bloody civil war had broken out.

The more I learned about Isaaq's heritage and background, the more I began to dread what was coming next in his story. It was like watching Edvard Munch slowly paint 'The Scream'. Long before it was finished, I knew the full picture was going to have a haunting impact.

Isaaq was nine years old when the genocide began. The Siad Barre regime carried out the systematic massacre of tens of thousands of members of Isaaq's clan. Burao was razed, with government soldiers going on a rampage through the town and killing civilians of all ages.

'They were pulled out, like this!' Isaaq said to me one day, clawing at straw in Rasher's pen. He grabbed handful after handful, throwing it violently onto the ground by his feet.

Witnessing his male relatives being dragged from their homes into the street had carved a deep and stirring memory.

It was a week later when Isaaq told the other men exactly what happened that day. All of the residents were in the TV lounge, taking part in a pool competition. A story had come up on the news about a shooting somewhere in America, which got them all talking. Isaac's memories must have been shaken to the fore again because he suddenly became very animated, his voice rising over all the others.

I was sunk almost without trace in the middle of one of the dilapidated sofas, having a tea break and reading some notes. I looked over to see Isaaq take aim very purposefully before firing a ball cleanly, and with tremendous force, into a pocket at the opposite end of the pool table.

'One by one, they shot my relatives dead. One by one, at point-blank range.'

He blasted another ball into a pocket, then another.

'What, not your brothers?' asked a support worker.

'No, not my brothers. My uncles, my older cousins. All of them.'

Putting down his cue, he leaned on the table with both arms, as if needing some support. He explained that he naively thought his brothers were 'spared' being shot because they were young – just 12, 13 and 15 years old.

'But then the bastards came back.'

Waiting to hear the fate of his siblings, the room stayed

still and silent, as if making a sound would somehow trample disrespectfully on Isaaq's memories.

I could hear my own heartbeat as I watched Isaaq solemnly stroke the skin on his neck then hold his hand across his heart. 'They pushed their heads forward and slit their throats, in front of me and my mother.'

In that moment it felt like the ceiling dropped, incomprehension and shock crashing down on everyone in the room.

Isaaq's mother hid him behind her baati skirt. He was small and skinny for a nine-year-old and she pleaded for his life, swearing he was only six and not of fighting age. Remarkably, her shrewd thinking saved his life.

Tens, if not hundreds, of thousands of others were not spared. The number of civilians killed in the massacre is estimated to be between 50,000 and 100,000, though it's claimed by locals the real figure could be as high as 200,000. I felt ashamed to have known so little about what has rightly been called a 'forgotten genocide'.

Burao was flattened and half a million Somalis fled across the border to Ethiopia. Isaaq, his mother and what remained of their extended family ended up as refugees, living in what became at the time the largest refugee camp in the world. There Isaaq was separated from his mother, apparently by accident. Weeks of searching proved fruitless. Not knowing what had become of her, he was eventually brought to England on a boat with other members of his clan who had willingly taken responsibility for him, knowing he had lost every other member of his family.

Upon arrival, his guardians were all held in a detention centre near Bristol, while ten-year-old Isaaq, having been born in the UK, was taken immediately into foster care.

Sitting with Gavin and me half an hour later, Isaaq moved on to the subject of his drug use. The reason for it might have seemed obvious. Surveys of adolescents receiving treatment for problematic substance use, for instance, have found that more than 70 per cent had a history of trauma. Isaaq himself had told me that at the start he took drugs to 'go to a different place for a few hours' and there was no doubting that, even by the age of ten, his eyes had seen things that anyone might want to anaesthetize themselves from the horror of. However, Isaaq's route into drugs was more complex than a straight cause-and-effect descent.

As the new boy at school in Bristol, it wasn't only the 'pirate' slur that made him feel alienated. He'd fallen behind the school curriculum and his fear of sudden loud noises and some of the playground games were noted by classmates. 'You're strange and you're darker than we are too,' one of the Black children told him. Isaaq couldn't understand the rejection because in Somali culture, everyone in your clan is your friend (at least until proven otherwise).

'In England, it seemed to be the other way round,' he said.

Lonely and displaced, 12-year-old Isaaq was easy prey for much older youths who hung around the school gates offering cigarettes and cans of beer. He was welcome in their group, they said, though what they didn't spell out was that their group was part of a criminal ring of drug dealers who were on the prowl for kids just like him. As a 'cleanskin', unknown to the police and therefore less likely to attract attention, Isaaq was the ideal new recruit. Within weeks, Isaaq had been groomed into 'running' – transporting drugs across the country and picking up dirty money for the dealers.

They call it 'county lines' today (a reference to the criminal gangs' phone networks), as if it's some new-fangled phenomenon. But organized-crime groups have been finding ways to expand their reach for centuries. It was harder to join the dots before mobile phones, but dealers have been pulling the strings of easily manipulated children (of all races and mostly, though not exclusively, boys) for as long as illicit substances have existed.

Isaaq told us how one of the other runners spent the drug money he collected instead of giving it to his boss. Isaaq was scared of what would happen next and even more terrified when he was told it was down to him to mete out the punishment.

'You want me to batter him? No, I don't want to. Why should I?'

'Because if you don't, we will do it to you, twice as hard.'

That was the start of Isaaq's training in violence, the next stage in his unsolicited criminalization. He was 14 when he started being noticed by the police and began picking up convictions. The courts saw a delinquent, not a trapped child, and he ricocheted between youth custody and children's homes.

No longer a 'cleanskin', Isaaq's usefulness to the group was over, in one way at least.

'They sent three men,' he said. 'I thought they were going to beat me up but they didn't.'

I remember the mixture of sickness and anger I felt when I heard this part of Isaaq's story. Instead of beating Isaaq up, two members of the drug gang pinned him down while a third injected him with heroin. The terror he was feeling morphed into a warm rush of detachment, as though his mind had uncoupled from his body and floated to the ceiling. If he had outlived his usefulness as a runner, they wanted to use him in other ways, not least as a customer with inflated drug debts to repay.

And Isaaq became a very good customer indeed. His missing eye, and the faded track marks on his arms and legs, were testament to that. He went back for more even after he had 'done his rattle', withdrawing from heroin in prison. It wasn't because he was physically addicted. 'I had no other life. I had a criminal record from 14. And sick though it was, drug users and drug dealers felt the closest thing I had to family.'

Isaaq was now 32 years old. All told, he had spent a decade of his life locked up. His longest prison stretch was for headbutting and kicking a paramedic who had been called to assist him one night when he'd been reported for 'acting bizarrely' on the street. He'd spent stints in psychiatric wards too. 'They pin you down and inject you with drugs there too,' he commented. 'The only difference is they are not your drugs, they are theirs.'

His latest offence was for kicking in a window in a shopping centre and resisting arrest. He explained that he was living in a bedsit after successfully completing a withdrawal programme and had been off all drugs, illicit or prescribed, for several months – a first since the age of 14.

'Why did you do that?'

'I was low. What prospects does a one-eyed Black ex-con have? I was on the verge of taking heroin or whatever shit I could find and I didn't have the energy for it again.'

Causing minor havoc in a shopping centre was Isaaq's ticket back to prison, a place where he felt at a lesser risk of relapsing. An overcrowded cell was the most ambitious future he could imagine.

As much as I would have liked to continue getting to know Isaaq and the other men at the project, my time there had to come to an end. I visited six months after my initial contract was over to deliver some more advanced staff training. Rasher was enormous and living in the grounds in her five-star accommodation. There were chickens running around too, as well as a couple of goats that had been abandoned by their previous owners. 'Their loss is my gain,' Isaaq declared.

By now, several more residents had moved in – still predominantly Black and mixed race – but the staff team (complete with a new deputy manager and a chef) was still lacking any diversity. The centre's location was always going to make it difficult to recruit BAME staff.

Building relations with the wider community had proved

an uphill struggle too and lack of inclusion in anything going on locally was an ongoing issue. There were no voluntary or work placements on offer nearby and for those who wanted to attend a local college, there wasn't one in striking distance. Some residents had started distance-learning courses online but Isaaq hopped on two buses and a train twice a week to study for a diploma in animal care.

I'd been made aware of Isaaq's ambitions a month prior to my last visit when I'd been asked to provide him with a reference and speak with the college's head of department, who was concerned about whether someone with a history of mental-health problems was 'safe to work with animals'.

Discrimination comes in many forms. As much as any illegal drug, it can be one of the reasons why some people 'go mad'; it maintains distress and can make recovery feel like wading through cement. In fact, it may result in some people never feeling fully 'recovered' at all because the discrimination they face has its tentacles in so many aspects of their lives.

I wasn't familiar with the term back then but working at the project had provided me with a valuable course in 'checking my privilege' – what social activist Peggy McIntosh calls 'an invisible package of unearned assets' that comes with being a member of a particular social group, such as being male, heterosexual, able-bodied, financially secure, born in a first-world country, living near a thriving city and so on. It doesn't mean that you don't struggle if you are in these groups but it acknowledges struggles that you are spared.

I'd certainly become more aware of my 'white privilege'

while at the project. Lesson one had taken place in the training room, when I realized I could go into any hair salon and they would be able to cut my hair. Lesson two had come when I reflected on the point that I'd been in hundreds of waiting rooms in my lifetime, never wondering if the cool reception I'd been given by those inside was something more than the usual wariness of strangers.

During the coronavirus lockdown in the UK in 2020, Jodie M Williams received a massive response when she asked people to share their experiences of white privilege. Her online exhibition *A Definition of White Privilege* – now also a book – includes hundreds of examples. For instance, white people have the privilege of being more likely to get access to psychological therapies for mental-health concerns and are less likely to be wrongfully stopped for shoplifting. White offenders have the privilege of not being given harsher sentences than others. White people can take it for granted that we can buy 'nude' plasters and tights that actually match our skin colour, or greetings cards and toys depicting people with the same colour skin as us. The list is long, and varied.

Through Isaaq and the other residents I had seen not just the unearned advantages my skin colour gave me but the unearned disadvantages their skin colour brought to them.

The biggest challenge that the drug-rehabilitation project faced wasn't in 'skilling up' the residents but in finding ways to level out the playing field that awaited them outside the project's walls.

*

Two years later, I met Gavin and Dougie for lunch. Gavin still worked at the unit, Dougie was a certified Pets as Therapy (PAT) dog, and there was some excellent news to share.

'I thought you'd like to see this.'

Gavin pushed a photograph across the table. It was a picture of Isaaq and Rasher, bathed in sunshine. Isaaq's hair was braided into neat cornrows and he was wearing a name badge on his smart green polo shirt. Rasher was in her grandest pen yet, with a piggy friend and being admired by a group of enthralled children.

Isaaq had not only received his diploma but had glowing recommendations from his tutors. After completing his rehab programme, he moved back to the Midlands where he'd been offered a job on a city farm, working with disadvantaged children. The staff and residents at the centre had voted unanimously that Rasher should go with him.

Isaaq had promised to keep in touch and send photographs as soon as they were settled in and he'd been true to his word.

'There's a note on the back,' Gavin said. 'I think you'll like it.'

I turned the photo over and smiled.

'This one-eyed Black ex-convict,' Isaaq had written, 'has prospects.'

How far we'd all come.

CHAPTER EIGHT
OUT OF THE HOT SEAT

Basil was at his most frenetic, hopping from one leg to the other, arms whirling and eyebrows wriggling like a couple of excited caterpillars.

'There you are! I need to talk to you!'

It'd be nice to get my coat off first, I thought, hastily stuffing my key fob back in my handbag as I shut the entrance door of Laurel House behind me.

It wasn't unusual to be ambushed like this. A lot could happen in the six-day space between my visits to the forensic step-down project and I was always expected to get up to speed quickly. Before I could blink, Basil was windmilling me through the staff office to his managerial quarters, a room that had once been a downstairs toilet in this formerly grand Edwardian house.

'We have a new resident,' he puffed. 'I need you to see him, urgently!'

I couldn't help but like Basil. He had been my colleague for nine years now. Despite being excruciatingly socially awkward most of the time, he had a good heart and was committed to doing his best for all the residents at the unit. He was the epitome of social-care workers, working round the clock for a low wage and precious little thanks, fired up by enthusiasm, goodwill and, in his case, a permanent state of the collywobbles.

'What's his name and what can you tell me about him?' I said slowly, trying to counter Basil's rising panic.

'Hayden, 29,' he volleyed back. Basil was stalking around his desk now, his words lightly echoing around the blue and white wave-patterned bathroom tiles that still covered the walls.

'He arrived two days ago from approved premises (what used to be known as probation hostels). He's been almost constantly in his room since. And when staff have been to check on him, he's been *curt*.'

'*Curt*? Why is he such a priority?'

Basil finally sat down and took a file from the top of his towering in-tray.

I unbuttoned my coat and helped myself to the only other seat while Basil started to give me more details. Hayden was out of prison on licence – in other words, he had been released early but with certain conditions, the breaking of which would see him go back to serve the rest of his term. He had been transferred to Laurel House from an approved premises in the Midlands where he'd been staying for the past three weeks.

'Why the move?' I asked.

'This is the issue, Kerry. The accommodation was near a primary school and Hayden started telling staff he was having thoughts of offending against children. The staff thought he was at immediate risk of abusing a child and, obviously, they wanted him moved quickly.'

Such was their hurry, in fact, they'd offloaded their worrying probationer to two members of our team on the side of a motorway near Stoke-on-Trent during morning rush-hour. It all seemed rather rash and so I asked the obvious question – had Hayden offended against children in the past?

'No,' Basil said, clicking his tongue on the roof of his mouth as he scanned the paperwork, 'though he has served time for attacking another vulnerable victim, namely an elderly woman with disabilities. He begged a residential worker to refer him to a psychiatrist who might prescribe anti-libidinal medication, which led to a discussion about whether a return to prison was appropriate.'

The crossover between those who target the elderly and those who target children for sexual assault is a deeply unpleasant topic that most people would prefer not to contemplate. Offenders willing to abuse those at the beginning of life are often willing to abuse those at the end, and vice versa. Because, as difficult as this may be to understand, frequently those who sexually attack children are not 'paedophiles' in the true or most commonly perceived sense of the word (just as those who sexually attack old folk are not 'gerontophiles'). These two groups of victims are the physically weakest and least able or likely to report; they're therefore equally 'attractive' prey in the mind of an abuser.

I looked Basil in the eye. 'So, you were saying, they considered sending Hayden back to prison?'

'Yes. Given the seriousness of what he described, a return to prison is still an option. His offender manager was shocked and decided he'd be better off here in the first instance, where he'll have a greater level of supervision and, of course, access to in-house psychiatry – and psychology.' With that Basil wafted one of his long arms out towards me, like an unwieldy conductor throwing the spotlight onto his orchestra for their applause.

'The psychiatrist isn't due until next Tuesday but we may need to call him out. Either way, I need you to see Hayden today. This morning, in fact.'

I frowned. 'What else can you tell me about his offence history?'

Basil fanned more paperwork across his desk. Hayden's offence had happened eight years previously, when he was 21 years old.

'His victim was a 78-year-old woman. His crime, I'm sorry to say, was rape.'

Basil cleared his throat and began reading from a summary.

'The victim lived alone in a development of one-bedroomed, specially adapted bungalows, managed by a charity as part of an independent-living scheme. She was blind, had learning difficulties and…'

I didn't need to hear what he said next.

In an instant, I'd been transported straight back to the late summer of 2004, my memories so finely etched I could almost taste the bitter coffee I drank when I arrived at the police station that morning.

*

I'd had a call at the crack of dawn, as was often the case in that era before police forces had their own staff trained in psychological techniques. By the time the clock struck 8.30am, I was already sitting in an airless office with the chief investigating officer and two plain-clothed police officers who both had specialist training in the investigation of rape and sexual offences, something of a rarity in the days before dedicated rape-investigation units were set up.

The first thing I noticed was that all three officers had the same look on their faces – one that told me they were not only sickened by the crime but absolutely determined to find the attacker. This was a case they *really* wanted to solve. The chief investigating officer wanted my help in planning the interviews with the victim. Any insight I might be able to provide to narrow down the pool of potential suspects would also be gratefully received.

I stirred two spoonfuls of sugar into my terrible coffee, my go-to move when the tea is just as awful and emergency caffeine is required. It usually makes the coffee just about palatable but this time it did nothing to disguise the nasty taste that stuck to my tongue as the officers swiftly brought me up to speed.

Had this been a TV police drama, the facts would probably have been drip-fed in tantalizing style over at least half an hour of television. As it was, the grim details were delivered wholesale, landing with cold thud after cold thud.

Lilian, known as Lily, had lived in her sheltered-housing bungalow for over 14 years. It was almost 4am that morning when she activated her Carelink emergency alarm; when the on-site community-support worker answered the call she found Lily in the bathroom, scared to death and wearing a nightie spotted with blood. 'The man,' she said, 'has done something to me, down there.'

The police were called and Lily was taken to hospital, where doctors concluded that the blood on her nightdress was from the rupturing of her hymen. Lily had previously been a virgin. Not that information regarding the nature, frequency or quality of sex, or lack of it, that a victim has had before being attacked makes a jot of difference. Nevertheless I remember the detail dialling my brain up from somewhere in the mid to high nineties to what felt like 200 per cent.

Lily had some bruising to her shoulders and inner thighs as well as small lacerations to her vagina. Swabs were taken and there was no evidence of seminal fluid (semen). Still, the medical staff were of the strong opinion that Lily had been raped.

So far, all that forensics had turned up was a partial shoe imprint on the lino of her entrance hall, which may or may not have been made by the perpetrator as he left through the front door of her property. The team was still at the scene and, as we spoke, all known sex offenders in the area were being checked up on. Lily, meanwhile, had been discharged from hospital and was being looked after by her younger brother and sister-in-law, who lived nearby.

Despite the early hour, the meeting was extremely lively. I'm sure the super-strength caffeine helped ignite us, but it was our united resolve to catch the man who'd carried out such a cowardly and deplorable attack that really put fire in our bellies. We all understood that if we caught him, we might stand a fighting chance of securing a conviction, thus protecting any other potential victims for at least the duration of his imprisonment. Disgracefully, this is the most elusive of outcomes in any rape case.

Currently, the prosecution of rape cases is at an all-time low. In the year up to March 2020, police recorded 55,259 rape complaints but only 2,102 of those cases were prosecuted, resulting in 1,439 convictions. It is a crushing set of statistics, amounting to what some justice campaigners have called the 'effective decriminalization of rape'.

Things were marginally better in 2004 but still nowhere even close to good enough. There has always been a reluctance to prosecute supposedly 'weak' rape cases, i.e. those that will challenge the decision-making of a jury, and the problem is that juries are heavily influenced by 'rape myths'. Dominic Willmott, a researcher at the University of Huddersfield, carried out a series of realistic simulations of rape trials and found that juries are reluctant to convict in cases that don't meet the public's 'psychological script' of what rape is.

Ninety per cent of rape victims are assaulted in their own home by someone they know and the go-to defence of perpetrators is to claim that consent was given. But, as Willmott puts it, large proportions of the public only recognize rape as a grubby stranger 'grabbing you in a bush and violently raping you'.

Lily, however, was not in the majority of victims, hitting as she did so many of the expectations that made her, from the public's (and therefore the CPS's) perspective, a 'credible' victim of rape.

Psychologist Jessica Eaton has compiled a hierarchy of characteristics that make up the 'perfect sexual violence victim', based on research in the UK from 2016 to 2018. It includes having no criminal record, not being intoxicated, not knowing the offender, not wearing provocative clothes, not being sexually active, having injuries to show and never having reported rape before. Sad to say, but short of being a nun who had fought her attacker tooth-and-nail in a dark alley, Lily could not have ranked much higher on the perfect rape victim score-o-meter.

'Let's not mess this one up,' was the phrase writ large in the shared thought bubble hanging in the muggy air at the police station that morning.

I didn't bother to tell Basil I'd worked on the original investigation. Eight years was a long time; it was a completely separate piece of work and, most importantly, I'd had nothing to do with Hayden himself. Besides, being the only psychologist in the building, I didn't have the luxury of being able to pass his case on.

I retreated to the staff office and began looking through Hayden's notes. A report detailing his participation in the prison-based Sex Offenders Treatment Programme (SOTP) immediately came to hand. Set up in 1991, the SOTP was the government's heavily rolled-out cognitive-behavioural group-therapy course for sex offenders serving sentences of four or more years (who, despite the lack of rape convictions, make up an ever-larger proportion of our bulging prison population, as sentences for sex offences have become progressively longer over the decades). The SOTP was the flagship of the offender treatment industry and forerunner of numerous similar interventions. In years to come, however, a damning piece of research would prove what anecdotal evidence had been telling those working with this group of offenders for a long time: it wasn't working and, not only that, it was in fact downright dangerous.

Hayden, it seemed, had been a star pupil of the SOTP, though it was noted he had 'initially found it difficult to come to terms with having committed the index offence'. *Oddly enough, a good sign*, I thought, as it's an indication of the ability to feel shame, at least. What 21-year-old man wouldn't want to fend off the acceptance that he'd raped a blind pensioner with learning difficulties, with all the connotations of deviancy and inadequacy that such a conviction holds?

The report elaborated that, 'During the first part of his sentence, he was keen to deny the offence or refused to discuss it. He has made much progress in this regard…he has acknowledged he had strong feelings of anger, powerlessness and sexual difficulties. These were magnified on the night of the offence following arguing with his girlfriend. Hayden has come to understand his actions as an attempt on his part to redress these emotions.'

The case had left everyone involved redressing some emotions. I'd like to say I'd never thought about Lily after Hayden's arrest, but that's not true. For a long time afterwards, I'd occasionally look at an elderly woman who reminded me of her, in a supermarket or at a zebra crossing, and have to blink away the image of a man forcing himself on her. Or a snippet from her evidence would pop into my head when I turned on the radio or sat in my garden with the sun on my face. Call it an occupational hazard, but for several months, there were nights when I dreamed there was someone in my house but I couldn't see them.

As I turned a page in the report I was reading, someone hammered so hard on the unlocked office door it fell wide open, spilling a gangly, flustered man into the room. His dark eyes were burning like dying bonfires. Grey crevices were carved in his wide, clammy forehead. It was Hayden.

'I'm sick in the head,' he announced as he began stalking haphazardly around the room. 'I want to see the psychiatrist. I need those drugs. When can I see the psychiatrist?'

How lovely to finally put a face to the name, I thought to myself sarcastically, *I've heard so much about you.*

Some forensic psychologists instruct their trainees that people in our profession cannot have emotions and that we must therefore learn to pack them into a tidy box that shall never be opened. This is nonsense. I'd worry that any psychologist who worked in this field and didn't periodically encounter flashes of rage, disgust, fear and every other human emotion was disturbingly desensitized. Emotional intelligence does not involve denying our automatic reactions. Rather, it is the ability to recognize and consciously greet them, then (in lightning speed) choose to respond to the situation based on our higher values and goals.

However, there is no denying that sometimes our moral outrage is so strong that it wins the battle and crashes into the room with us. It had happened when I'd interviewed Adele in prison and now, confronted with Hayden, it was testing me to the limit once again.

'I know who you are,' I wanted to whisper. 'I know *what* you are.' The strength of my reaction at seeing this man took me by surprise. What I was feeling was unfamiliar – it was a cold, hard contempt.

So much for thinking this was totally separate from the work I did on the case eight years earlier.

In hindsight, I can see that there was more to my reaction to Hayden than simply my history with the investigation. Though I didn't recognize it at the time, at this point in my career I'd started on the long journey towards burnout. Austerity, the butcher's knife that was taken to government services to eliminate budget deficits after the global financial crisis of 2008, meant the wide portfolio of contracts and referrals I'd enjoyed juggling had started being trimmed away like fat on a tenderloin. Funding cuts to courts, police, prison and probation services would see me explaining to my private-practice colleagues, who were also my friends, that I no longer had enough work to share with them. My one day a week at Laurel House was my last remaining regular contract and it would soon be put out to tender, only to disappear in a puff of penny-pinching smoke. Meanwhile, what remained of my once-varied caseload had filtered into what felt like a constant drone of trial and pre-sentence reports requested in only the most dire of circumstances – murder, manslaughter and child sexual-abuse cases. So many child sexual-abuse cases and yet only the tip of an iceberg.

Eyes that blur with seeing too much, a mind that becomes paralysed by knowing too much. Vicarious trauma, emotional overload – call it what you like, I was drawing on the plastic inner warrior in my tea cupboard more than usual. The enormity of the tragedy contained in even one case can linger and feel overwhelming. The filthy, unrelenting tide of violence and child abuse I was swimming in was being gradually absorbed.

'I can't cope any longer with these thoughts in my head. I don't want to touch any kids. I need that medication today. I need to see the psychiatrist!'

Here was a fellow human being in front of me, asking for help. He felt overwhelmed too and yet, when I listened to Hayden's desperate demands, I felt numb. The first sign of 'compassion fatigue', described by trauma specialist Charles Figley as 'the cost of caring', was setting in.

'I need the drugs! I want it to stop!' I could hear Hayden loud and clear but when I looked at him, I couldn't fully see him. My mind was still lodged in 2004 and I was thinking of what Lily had told the police.

*

Back in the land of crime fiction, the witness is interviewed at home or in a hospital bed by a detective who opens his notebook, licks the top of his pen and then proceeds with all the panache of a wasp at a barbecue. Questions are rattled off, seemingly without any preparation, structure or consideration of the impact on the individual answering them. That may have been common decades ago, but not in 2004. And certainly not when the witness account may be all the police have to work with and is coming from a person like Lily – terrified and in need of support.

It took the 1991 Orkney Child Abuse Investigation and the Clyde Report of 1992 to officially identify a serious lack of training for interviewers of vulnerable witnesses. The Memorandum of Good Practice (MOGP) on how to interview children for criminal proceedings was created to address these shortcomings. Fantastic progress, but it didn't cater for other vulnerable members of our communities, including adults with learning disabilities. The MOGP was eventually reassessed and improved upon, resulting in the 2002 'Achieving Best Evidence: Guidance for vulnerable or intimidated witnesses, including children'.

One of the main issues when interviewing a vulnerable person is not the amount of information they know but what fails to be correctly teased out. Our priority was working out how to get every scrap of useful information from Lily without adding to her distress.

There was a heck of a lot to think about. Lily had both physical and mental challenges to consider. She would be providing predominantly ear-witness rather than eye-witness testimony and we had to gain some further understanding of how her learning difficulties might make communication more of a struggle for her. If the case ever got to a trial, it was unlikely that anyone would want to put Lily through the torment of taking the stand, an intensely stressful job under the best of circumstances. The videos of Lily's police interviews might therefore be used as evidence in chief and, as such, they needed to be meticulously planned and flawlessly executed. We also needed to act quickly, while Lily's recollections of events were fresh and uncontaminated in her mind.

The plans I drew up with David and Val, the two specialist officers, were heavily based on the 'Enhanced Cognitive Interview' technique. The original Cognitive Interview method is derived from ideas first discussed by Frederic Bartlett in his 1932 book *Remembering,* the principle being that our memories are stored as a network of associations (rather than unconnected events) which can be accessed in a number of ways.

The Cognitive Interview uses four main strategies to help interviewees retrieve knowledge: 'mental reinstatement of context' (helping them to think back to where they were, how they felt, what the weather was like and so on); 'report everything' (no information is irrelevant, so the report of any and all detail is encouraged); 'recall events in different temporal orders' (asking interviewees to start at the middle or end and work backwards, for instance) and 'change perspective' (asking interviewees to describe the events from the perceived point of view of any other people present).

The Enhanced Cognitive Interview was brought in after police complained the original model wasn't 'socially supportive' of witnesses. It improved the amount of information reported but was not the kindest approach (for example, asking the victims of serious assaults to look at photographs of the crime scene as 'reinstatement of context' can be nothing short of cruel). As a result, several extra elements were added, including a chatty, rapport-building phase and more consideration of how the interview process would be experienced by the witness. This was exactly the model we needed to tailor around Lily.

Needless to say, it's a much more time-consuming piece of work than a standard interview. We sat for a day and a half solid, in an office that smelt of biscuits and Eau Sauvage, thrashing out the interview strategy in fine detail. It is always difficult to slot yourself into an already well-established team (particularly as a psychologist, because we are often viewed as only one step in the food chain above psychics or people who ring up to discuss their 'helpful' theories after watching a YouTube documentary on a cold case). However, by the second morning, I realized that I'd been accepted when David and Val started referring to me as 'Ginge'.

While we were hard at work, another officer was dispatched to talk to Lily's brother and sister-in-law and the community-support worker at her housing development, who provided lots of valuable information about Lily's lifestyle, interests and the nature of her disabilities. Her attacker still at large, we were ready to talk to Lily herself by the afternoon of day two.

Val took the lead in the interview as I watched a live feed on an old Sony Trinitron TV in a next-door room along with the chief investigating officer, a man with apparently no name as I'd only heard him referred to as 'Chief'. The walls were paper thin, so we spoke to each other in low murmurs while he chain-smoked out of the window.

Lily had fine, shoulder-length white curls and was dressed in a well-loved summer smock and hand-knitted cardigan. She was guided into the room by her sister-in-law, who held her hand, stroking it tenderly and not letting go as they took their places on a two-seater sofa.

'Poor old dear,' tutted Chief, blowing a smoke ring in my direction. 'I can't get my head around any sicko who'd molest an old lady like that.'

I drew a line in the air, breaking up the smoke ring with my pen. People find it hard to understand why an offender would commit a sexual assault of any kind against someone who doesn't fit the stereotype of a sexually desirable person, but age offers no protection against sexual victimization. Rape is predominantly about wielding power, not fulfilling sexual desire.

Sexual assaults against pension-age women are not as uncommon as the public imagines, though there's a dearth of data and first-person accounts to prove it. Taboo and denial around older people having *any* kind of sex, consenting or otherwise, are major inhibitors to disclosure, discussion and analysis. You would expect the rape of elderly victims to be worthy of particular study but it is an area that is all but ignored. Social worker Malcolm Holt collected hundreds of anecdotal accounts of sexual abuse of elderly women, over 55 per cent of whom were abused by their sons. Another rare study found that 3.1 per cent of sexual-offence victims in a rural area of England over a five-year period were over the age of fifty-five. But wider-ranging figures don't exist because, for reasons nobody seems to know, the Home Office does not categorize its rape statistics by age and, until recently, the Crime Survey for England and Wales only asked those under the age of 59 questions about 'intimate violence'.

The real rarity of Lily's case was that it had come to the attention of police in the first place. She had shown courage in agreeing to be here just days after the attack and I was pleased to see that she looked remarkably relaxed, smiling and putting out her hands to briefly hold that of each officer as Val began the introductions.

The first phase of the interview was taken up talking to Lily about the keep-fit class she attended and her love of audio books, things her relatives and carers had said were important to her. Lily even managed to laugh when Val told her that she'd once fallen flat on her face in an exercise class and had never gone back.

'What have you listened to lately? I wish I had more time to read.'

'*The Graveyard Book* and *The Host*. I like ghost stories.'

'Oh, they'd scare me. What is *The Graveyard Book* about, then?'

Small talk in any other situation, crucial groundwork in this scenario. We'd been told that Lily had more than adequate verbal communication skills, as long as sentences were kept short and clear. Counting her words (as David would be doing in the interview room) told me that Lily used no more than ten words per sentence on average, so that would serve as our guide when asking questions.

'Do you know why you are here today, Lily?' asked Val.

'Because a man came into my house. He did something to me.'

'That's right. In a little bit I am going to ask you to tell us everything you can remember about what happened. Try as hard as you can, really think about what happened the night the man came in. We want you to tell us everything you can, even if you only remember bits of it, don't leave anything out.'

Val began to prompt Lily to close her eyes and think about where she was just prior to 'the man' entering her home, reassuring her that she was safe now. What could she hear? What could she feel? In her own time and at her own pace, Lily began providing some really useful information.

It had been a warm night and Lily had been sitting just outside the front of her bungalow in her nightie and dressing gown. She recalled the sound of her wind chime – a birthday present from her neighbour. When it began to get cooler, she went inside and turned the radio on.

'It was playing a horrible noise, so I turned it down. And then I heard him come in. He pushed me. He was on top of me.'

Lily thought long and hard, her sister-in-law still stroking her hand intermittently, letting her know she was doing well.

'Take your time, Lily,' David said.

Lily struggled with the language to describe the rape but said enough to make it clear what had happened.

'And he kept saying things to me. I didn't know what he meant. I didn't know what he wanted me to do.'

There was a long pause. 'What he wanted you to do?' repeated Val.

'He wanted me to put my hands on his back. He said, "Use your nails."'

Having no sexual experience Lily didn't understand what he was asking or why, and she had remained frozen, gripping tight to her sofa. Eventually, the man started to apologize to her, saying to her, 'It isn't you...I'm sorry, do you mind? I'm sorry, tell me it was good.'

Though Lily didn't have any grasp of what the man was saying sorry for, it seemed from her description that he was apologizing for and seeking reassurance about his sexual performance, and possibly for the fact he wasn't able to ejaculate.

'He said, "You should lock your door." I think he went then. I remember listening to Robbie Williams. But I was too scared to get up.'

Lily looked exhausted already, so we took a break from

the interview while David and I compared our notes. The questioning crucial to the investigation hadn't yet begun, but a picture was already emerging. The bizarre but not altogether unique 'conversation' that Lily was reporting was one I've heard variations of numerous times, with offenders desperate to coerce a fantasy of intimacy from their victim, to convince themselves that they are sexually competent and their victim is somehow complicit in the process. Apologizing, demanding participation from a victim and the less overtly aggressive type of activity seen here are the trademarks of an anxious, socially unskilled offender – one who is driven to exert control over a victim to reassure himself of his masculinity. Men who fit this type are often called 'power assurance rapists' or 'gentleman rapists' by academics. The latter phrase incorporates two words that, if you ask me, don't deserve to be used in the same sentence together.

As interesting as it is, a glimpse into the psychological state of the offender doesn't bring anything particularly useful to the table in an investigation like this. If we were ever to find who did this to Lily, we needed much more to go on.

Val and David started their questioning in earnest, using the strategies we'd planned to jog Lily's memory. They began with the radio programme and worked from there. After a series of open-ended questions, it wasn't long before we'd learned that Lily had been listening to her local radio's nightly request show. She couldn't tell us the time it started but she could tell us what songs she remembered hearing.

Chief stubbed his cigarette out on the aluminium window frame and left the room for five minutes to assign someone the task of tracking down a recording of the show. With the help of the radio station, it took only a small amount of digging to figure out that the 'horrible noise' that Lily had referred to was an advert for a local nightclub, one that signed off with the cry of a tropical bird. The police were then able to draw up an accurate timeline of when the attack took place, something that Lily hadn't been able to tell us and even the best of witnesses often misjudge. It was just after 9.36pm, in fact, when she went to turn the volume down on her radio and just 21 minutes later that Robbie Williams's 'Something Beautiful' started playing.

There were many things that Lily could not tell us and Val instructed her not to guess at. It was a 'man's voice' was all that Lily could say, her learning difficulties preventing her from extrapolating an accent or approximate age as others might. Similarly, Lily wasn't able to estimate the perpetrator's size or build, other than to say, 'He was very big and strong,' as any victim might perceive an unknown attacker.

Still, there was much that Lily *could* tell us. She recalled a rough, cold scratch on the right side of her face. Working backwards from the Robbie Williams song, she reiterated that 'He told me, "You should lock your door." Then I heard the door shut.'

'Can you remember anything he said before that?'

'He said I had to keep myself safe. He said, "Don't just rely on your Carelink alarm."'

A bit of self-deception-cum-victim-blaming disguised as advice. Abhorrent, given that it had taken a mere 21 minutes under his control for Lily to possibly never feel safe again. But the information contained in that statement was an investigator's dream.

The attacker's knowledge of the specific alarm system Lily had fitted in her bungalow wasn't the only important clue he had left. The lack of semen was not by clever design. There was nothing in Lily's account to suggest he had used a condom and he'd apologized for not being able to ejaculate. Add to this the fact that he instructed Lily to scratch his back, risking valuable DNA evidence lodging in her fingernails, and it was clear this offender was less forensically aware than your average *CSI* viewer. Most offenders with previous convictions for sexual or serious offences might have learned the hard way to avoid leaving crucial evidence. Therefore, the list of convicted rapists and serious sex offenders living in the area was unlikely to prove fruitful and the police could de-prioritize that line of enquiry.

An offender's 'profile' very often presents itself quite easily – a modicum of investigative nous and a dose of common sense are the only skills required to see it. Based on that and rough statistical data, what we knew of the attacker's behaviour pointed to him being someone young, possibly with a minor record of drugs offences but less likely for burglary (given that nothing was taken from Lily's home, as is often the case in the rare event of a stranger assaulting a woman in her own home) and living locally. Clearly, the fact that the rapist knew about the Carelink alarm Lily had installed in her bungalow pointed to him being someone very close to home indeed.

It didn't take the police long to zero in on Hayden, the tall, square-jawed boyfriend of the community-support worker who lived in a bungalow on the far edge of the site – the same young woman who had responded to Lily's initial emergency alarm call.

Hayden's only previous contact with police had been when he had been found smoking cannabis when he was 17, which hadn't led to any formal action. He was spoken to on day four of the investigation and immediately drew attention to himself by denying any knowledge whatsoever of the assault, which was a misguided strategy given that his girlfriend had been pulled out of bed to find Lily and had already told police she had discussed it with him. Meanwhile, she was unable to provide Hayden with an alibi. They'd argued that night and he'd stormed off at around 9pm, not returning to her home until after pub closing time. The landlord of the pub where he claimed to have spent the evening was adamant that they hadn't served him until last orders.

Forensics matched a man's trainer found in the hallway of the girlfriend's bungalow with the imprint on Lily's hall floor. The clothes Hayden had been wearing on the night of the assault included a T-shirt with a right-side zipped pocket on the chest, which would account for the cold scratch Lily felt to her face. Add to that there was the 'golden nugget' of evidence: a tiny amount of saliva found on the top of Lily's nightie matched with the DNA sample taken from their suspect by police. Nonetheless, Hayden pleaded not guilty to the rape. A unanimous jury disagreed.

Does a single act define a person? Is it right to forever call someone a 'rapist' if on one day, out of the over 7,655 days of their life, they choose to rape another person? Possibly. Or maybe that is ill-considered, over-simplified.

This man is more than just his offending behaviour, I told myself. *You know what he did back then but you don't know who he is now.*

'You must be Hayden. I'm Kerry, I'm the psychologist here and was planning to come and talk with you today.'

There was something about Hayden's demeanour that helped me to talk myself round and refocus. When he finally hurled himself into the chair on the opposite side of my desk, I could see not just irritability but abject misery in his eyes.

'You've got to help me. Please! I can't deal with this much longer,' he pleaded.

Compassion fatigue or not, I could see that I wasn't the only one who'd almost reached a tipping point that day.

'I've been told that there's medication that can help me.'

'Well, I understand that you've been asking for antilibidinal medication. I can't prescribe that, you'd have to speak to our psychiatrist, but I can tell you that they act by lowering testosterone levels.'

Hayden was listening intently now, nodding his head.

'They decrease sexual interest and arousal, but there are lots of side-effects that you have to be aware of too.'

'I don't care, as long as they get these fucking thoughts out of my brain,' he said, banging the heel of his hand on his temple.

It's very unusual for a man who's just been released from prison – and a near eight-year stretch at that – to be insisting so dramatically and vociferously that he wanted to be 'chemically castrated'.

'Well, antilibidinal drugs are never the full answer,' I continued. 'They would only be considered as part of a bigger care plan to help you avoid future reoffending. It's usually psychological work that...'

I didn't get to the end of my sentence. 'I've done all the groups and stuff in prison, it's what put this shit in my head. I'm not doing any more of that now,' he countered, his voice rising.

'Alright, we have lots of other psychology options that we can talk about. I can see from your file here what you've taken part in before.'

Before Hayden could take that in, a couple of support workers came through the door. 'Don't mind us,' one said spryly. 'Everything alright?' the other asked, suddenly reading the room.

'Fine,' I said, because, as things go in this environment, enough was under control.

I suggested to Hayden we go and sit in the lounge area next door, where at this time of day we'd have a better chance of talking uninterrupted. He bobbed his head in agreement and, after I'd locked his notes back into the filing cabinet, he followed me silently out of the room.

We sat opposite each other, Hayden on the sofa and me on a stained and sour-smelling armchair that I didn't want to contemplate too deeply. *Another case of compassion fatigue*, I thought, slipping a crust-thin cushion under my bottom. There was no chance of Hayden sitting comfortably either. Perched on the edge of his seat and tapping his feet faster than Ann Miller in a classic cinema musical, he was clearly in a pronounced state of arousal, but it wasn't sexual arousal.

'I need that medication,' he was repeating, his jaw bones grinding.

'The medication should only be prescribed to those who would actually benefit from it, that means men who have hyper-sexual arousal – feel always turned on – or are preoccupied with sexual matters,' I told him. I was aware that I sounded like I was giving an educational lecture on pharmacological approaches to sex-offending risk but Hayden should have the facts about what he was demanding. 'That's not something that I've read in your SOTP summary,' I went on. 'Or in your Structured Assessment of Risks and Needs that was relevant to your offence.'

I had not come across a single mention of abnormal sexual arousal in Hayden's documents. What had struck me while reading them was that Hayden appeared to have been absolutely honest during his prison psychology sessions about what he had done to Lily. His ultimate analysis, and that of the other SOTP group members and facilitators, was that he'd had 'strong feelings of anger, powerlessness and sexual *difficulties*', including erectile dysfunction, that were magnified on the night of the rape by arguing with his girlfriend.

'Does hyper-arousal sound like what is happening to you now?'

'I'm not sure. I'm just so scared…'

'So the thoughts are scary, Hayden? Can you tell me more about that?'

'I'm scared of what they mean. They won't go away. They come to me when I'm in my room, on my own, just watching television or something. I'll do anything not to do those things!'

'It's reassuring that you don't want to act on these thoughts. It sounds like they are upsetting. Do you find them sexually arousing?'

He flashed me a look of horror and astonishment. 'No. I find them disgusting.'

There was a pause as Hayden relaxed tapping his feet a little. He seemed lost in thought.

'But I'm scared because I did that, didn't I? I did that to a blind old lady. I know what I'm capable of.'

I must admit that the uncharitable voice in the back of my mind wormed its way to the front again. *Yes, I know what you are capable of as well.*

'I was disgusted with myself then too,' he continued. 'That night, I ran away shouting to myself, "You bastard, you bastard." If I did that, maybe I could do it to a kid? I could, couldn't I? I'm a sick bastard, aren't I?'

Anxiety was rising in his voice. His argument made sense but the more I listened to him, the less I shared his fears, or those of the staff at the project, about the likelihood of him harming children. People who intend to abuse only rarely announce it and it is highly unusual for them to beg for antilibidinal drugs.

'Help me understand more about these thoughts. Describe as much as you can about them.'

'It's like a broken film starts playing in my head, whether I want it to or not. I can't stop it.' He hunched his shoulders forwards and dropped his head over his jangling thighs as he described disjointed pictures, words and the sensation of hands on bodies, a sharp pain.

'I don't want them there!' he shouted, hitting his hand on the side of his head again, as though trying to physically knock the unwelcome visitors out. 'I don't want these thoughts in my head.'

The movement in his legs suddenly travelled up the whole of his body. It was as if he'd been plugged into the mains and now his whole body was shaking like an electric blender. Moments later, he juddered to a halt and then froze. He was holding his breath and his eyes were staring at the coffee table in front of him, though I don't think he was looking at the white circles stained into the once-polished wood.

'Hayden, Hayden?' I said cautiously. 'That's right, look at me, breathe with me.'

I put my hand on my chest, letting out a slow, exaggerated breath to the count of five.

Hayden wasn't having thoughts indicative of wanting to sexually abuse a child, he was having flashbacks.

Over the next two hours, Hayden told me that 'the thoughts' had started to emerge during the six months plus he'd spent on the Sex Offenders Treatment Programme in prison. Asking him about his participation in the accredited course – the successful completion of which is the golden ticket to parole for many – seemed to open a door that let in just enough light for Hayden to start seeing more clearly what was taking place in his own mind.

'Some of the lads did SOTP just to look good,' he told me. 'Loads do it. Just say what they want you to say, cheat the assessments by exaggerating a few things at the beginning, then tell the truth at the end so it looks like you've improved. But that's not why I did it. I took it seriously.'

One of the key features of the SOTP was the notorious 'hot seat'. Each inmate would have to take their turn in the seat, describing their crimes in painstaking, extended detail. The idea was that other members of the group would feel and express repugnance and challenge the 'deviant' attitudes and beliefs of the person in the spotlight. To make this more likely, SOTP groups were deliberately made up of a mix of different kinds of offender; those in Hayden's group, for example, had been jailed for everything from the sexual assault of women and teenage boys to the rape and murder of pre-school age children.

'I didn't want to go back after I'd done my hot seat.' Hayden was trembling as he spoke, clearing his throat as it constricted with the recollection. 'I couldn't stand listening to it all. Or watching it. Some of them were getting off on it, you knew they'd be fantasizing about it all later.'

Former prison psychologist Robert A Forde, one of the SOTP's most long-standing critics, points out that trying to alter people's behaviour patterns by attacking their attitudes and beliefs can be seriously counter-productive. It provokes a defensive reaction that reinforces the mindset that it seeks to eliminate. He highlighted the striking similarities in the SOTP's methods to those used in the early days of communist China to 'brainwash' westerners who had been found to be creating political propaganda. They were imprisoned and similarly encouraged to challenge each other's points of view, with their progress measured by how willing they were to reform their own thought processes as well as by their success in changing their cellmates' state of mind. Those dissidents who were lucky enough to be returned to the West often came home with problems that would today be viewed as post-traumatic stress. Moreover, although the westerners improved their understanding of the Chinese point of view while undergoing their 're-education' (or at least, did their best to look like they had), as soon as they were back in their old environment, surrounded by like-minded people, they quickly reverted to their original beliefs. As Forde states, 'It is a truism that those who do not learn from history's mistakes are condemned to repeat them.'

'Sometimes I feel like I'm back there,' Hayden said. 'I tried making excuses not to go but the prison staff always persuaded me. It would have counted against me if I missed sessions, they said. I didn't want to fail the programme. One week, I felt like I just froze and left my body.'

'It sounds like that was a pretty harrowing and significant week for you.'

He nodded and took a sip from the glass of water I'd gone to get him. 'There's something,' he said, purposefully stopping to take another sip, as if stalling for time. Slowly placing the glass down, he gripped his knees tightly. As he did so the look of anxiety on his face seemed to distort into one of fear. 'I don't know if I'm allowed to say it. I don't want you to think I'm playing at being the victim.'

'You have my permission to say whatever you feel is important.'

'When I froze, it was like I was paralysed. I couldn't run off, I couldn't think straight. I could feel his hands on me and I felt sick.'

'His hands on you?' I repeated, not quite understanding.

'Not the one in the hot seat. *His* hands.'

Hayden, it emerged, had been a boy of 12 when he was sexually abused by a 17-year-old cousin who had come to stay during the school holidays, sharing Hayden's bedroom.

'I never told anyone; my family would never have believed me. I just wanted to forget it but it was the opposite. I couldn't stop thinking about it and it was like it followed me, always. Everywhere.'

Hayden's first attempt to discuss his childhood abuse was with a prison psychologist who apparently told him that it was 'not relevant' in terms of his treatment. I can only assume that what he or she was *trying* to say was that there is no direct or predestined pathway between sexual victimization in childhood and becoming an abuser. And that is absolutely true.

There's an opening scene in Glen Duncan's novel *I, Lucifer* where the devil is tempting a priest to sexually assault a choirboy, nine-year-old Emilio. He congratulates himself on the fact that Emilio's victimization had laid some pretty useful foundations in him, commenting, 'That's the beauty of my work, it's like pyramid selling.' The devil was overly confident. Sexual abuse does not work in anything like such a simple cause-and-effect way. If it did, you would first have to ask why it is that women (who in the UK are three times more likely to have been subjected to sexual abuse before the age of 16 than men) are therefore not the main perpetrators of sex crime.

Approximately 1 per cent of men in England and Wales are convicted of a sexual offence at some point in their lifetime (although, as we have seen, many more dodge any legal consequences). Around 10 per cent of men who have been damaged by sexual abuse as boys go on to become convicted sex offenders. So, pulling those figures together means that childhood victimization makes men around ten times more likely to later join the ranks of perpetrator, but also that 90 per cent of sexually abused men will never offend in this way. Being the victim of early sexual abuse is never an excuse for victimizing others. It can be highly relevant to understanding the pathway to sexual offending in *some* individuals but is only ever a sharp-edged shard of the whole picture.

Humans are 'meaning-making' creatures in that we try to create solid and usable sense out of the confusion of life baggage we collect and carry around. There was nobody in 12-year-old Hayden's life he felt close enough to talk to or certain enough of their response to be able to confide in. He was on his own, floundering with the question 'Why me?'

'I didn't know what it meant about who I was. For ages, I thought it must have made me gay or something.'

Despite feeling frightened and repulsed, Hayden had briefly experienced an erection while being abused. It was purely a physical reaction but he couldn't understand why his body had betrayed him that way, exacerbating his doubts about his sexual orientation. In time, all of his anxieties converged into a deep fear that others would notice his 'lack of masculinity'.

'I'd panic in case my dad noticed something different about me. He'd have gone mad if he thought I'd been with a boy.' He was also worried that another boy would somehow spot his unwilling 'gayness'. 'What if a lad saw it and tried to touch me?'

Hayden told me he looked at porn from the age of 13 in an effort to reaffirm his heterosexuality. Not surprisingly, it didn't help matters – pornography never gave anyone a balanced view of sexual relationships or performance. When you looked beyond the furrowed brow, slick skin and angry eyes, you could see that Hayden was blessed with handsome looks. As a teenager, he'd had no trouble attracting the girls and, in his rush to become sexually active, he pressurized them into having sex with him. However, far from quelling his worries, his fumbling encounters failed to match up to the manufactured images of hardcore porn he'd pored over. He was left 'feeling ratty, panicky…like I needed to have sex with girls to prove myself but would never be good enough, man enough, for them'.

On the night that he'd raped Lily, Hayden was convinced that his girlfriend was going to dump him. As he walked through the supported-housing estate en route to the pub, he made up his mind to find a woman, any woman, to have sex with. Lily was a far less intimidating figure than the girls he was attracted to. When he saw her walking back into her bungalow as the sun set on her small patch of front garden, he followed her inside.

When I told Basil I didn't think Hayden was an immediate threat to children, his caterpillar eyebrows drew together as though in a fearful embrace.

'But he's saying that he wants to assault them.'

'He hasn't said anything of the sort. If you listen carefully, he is saying that he is frightened of the thought of assaulting children. Because the idea is abhorrent to him.'

I remember thinking I was glad I hadn't encountered Hayden when I was a younger and more inexperienced psychologist because I could have all too easily fallen into the same trap of accepting his interpretation of his thoughts at face value. He would have been left alone to wrestle with the same feelings of powerlessness, anger and confusion that, in the past, had led to him being a danger to women.

Basil looked sceptical and concerned but he let me continue.

I explained Hayden's ordeal during the hot-seat sessions of the SOTP, how taking part had triggered a reliving of his own abuse at the hands of his cousin and my belief that the thoughts that were repeatedly gate-crashing his mind were flashbacks, created from knotted-together residue of trauma that he'd lived through himself, or from the recounting of others' offences.

This was clearly not what Basil was expecting to hear. 'So you can develop intrusive thoughts and pictures of things that have happened to others, just from hearing about it?' he asked.

'Oh yes,' I replied, knowing that I could personally vouch for that. Basil still looked somewhat dubious.

My morning with Hayden hadn't exactly resulted in a lightbulb moment either – he was far too traumatized to process all that we had discussed in the flick of a switch – but he'd started to consider that there might be a different meaning to be made of what was happening to him. By the end of our marathon conversation, a glimmer of relief had crossed his eyes, some stillness finally starting to settle around him. All in all, a good morning's work.

I continued to work with Hayden for the next four months, at which point my contract at Laurel House ran out. The more time I spent with him, the more I was convinced that he hadn't 'failed' the SOTP, but the SOTP had failed him. Although luckily not as spectacularly as it had failed others.

Naomi Bryant was raped and strangled in Winchester in 2005 by SOTP graduate Tony Rice, nine months after he was released on licence from a life sentence imposed for three rapes and sexual assaults. The coroner at her 2011 inquest said the case was 'a wake-up call for those involved in offender management'.

It would be several years after I worked with Hayden that the diamond in the crown of the offending behaviour treatment industry would be exposed as nothing more than costume jewellery. In 2017, the SOTP was quietly, and without explanation, scrapped (although programmes based on the SOTP still run to this day in some forensic hospital services). At the same time, an embarrassing study – dating back to 2012 – had been uploaded without fanfare into the bowels of a government website, where former Justice Minister Liz Truss no doubt hoped it would stay. An election was looming and nobody wanted voters to be aware that the Ministry of Justice had been sitting on a costly failure, but that is exactly what they had been doing.

The large-scale study had compared men who had completed the Sex Offenders Treatment Programme with untreated sex offenders over an average of 8.2 years after their release from prison. The number who were convicted of another sex offence was low compared to other types of offending – 8 per cent for untreated men but 10 per cent for those who had 'successfully' graduated from the SOTP. Participation in the psychological treatment resulted in a small but significant *increase* in risk. In human terms, one that equates to 20 new victims for every 1,000 men who once took their place in the hot seat.

When I bid Hayden and the project goodbye, he was no longer plagued by disturbing thoughts of child abuse but was ready to work on developing his understanding of what healthy and satisfying sexual relationships look like.

Almost ten years have passed since then and I have it on good authority he has never reoffended.

CHAPTER NINE

BLOOD, SWEAT AND FEARS

The peace of the evening was shattered as the woman charged out of her front door and began calling to all the little girls playing in the cul-de-sac.

'Come, come!' she implored, her dark eyes flitting between the clusters of children making the most of the fading six o'clock sunshine. 'I need all the girls. All the girls! Gather round, come, come! All of you!'

Several of the younger children – girls aged around seven and eight – reluctantly stopped their games and walked towards her. Aleena, a 46-year-old former teacher was familiar to them. She had lived in the detached house at the top of their close for many years. The curtains of her house were pulled tightly closed on that particular late afternoon. And although Aleena looked oddly intense, gesturing to the girls in an increasingly exaggerated manner to come over to her, her urgency obliged them to do as they were told.

'She's off her rocker,' one of the older boys hissed to his little sister. 'Stay away from her. I'm going to tell Mum.'

As he laid down his scooter a yelp of alarm shot through the muggy air. Looking up, the boy saw that the woman had blood running from the palms of her hands. Not only that, she had pressed a glistening ruby spot of it onto the forehead of a small auburn-haired girl, who was standing stock still with tears welling up in her eyes as she took in the startled faces of her friends.

'I need to see blood,' Aleena had begun to chant quietly. 'I need to see blood.'

The boy grabbed his sister and darted to his front door. Other children started screaming and crying, scattering in panic, only heightening Aleena's agitation.

'I need to see blood,' she repeated, now running at the children with outstretched arms, drops of blood peppering the warm pavement slabs.

By the time the mums and dads had rushed into the street, Aleena had managed to seize several other girls, holding them by one arm for long enough to daub their faces with the red liquid too. It wasn't immediately obvious to the parents where the blood had come from. Inevitably, all hell broke out.

The adults snatched their children up and circled Aleena. With her laboured breathing and blood now smeared down the front of her peach-coloured blouse she looked nothing short of the archetypal madwoman to them.

'What the fuck is wrong with you?' one mother demanded to know.

After a moment spent taking in the angry sea of faces, Aleena began hurling insults back, loudly berating the parents for allowing their daughters to play unsupervised in the street. 'You don't do anything about these girls!' she shrieked, waving an admonishing finger. 'I need to see blood. I have to see blood!'

One of the mothers threatened to punch her in the mouth if she didn't shut up. She might well have carried out her threat had Aleena's husband not cut through the crowd, apologizing profusely as he ran forward and wrapped his arms tightly around his wife. It was more like a restraining motion than a hug and she tried, uselessly, to shrug him off. As she did so, Aleena didn't look at her husband. Instead, her eyes were still scouring the cul-de-sac.

'I need to see blood,' she repeated weakly. 'Where are all the girls? I need to see blood.'

Meanwhile, the parents continued shouting, some of them making increasingly hostile threats and calling Aleena names – 'nut job' and 'psycho' being probably the least offensive of them.

'You need to sort her out!' one woman shouted, prodding her finger at Aleena's husband. 'We're not putting up with this! She needs locking up, the freak.'

'I'm sorry,' Aleena's husband said, looking around at his neighbours. 'She doesn't know what she is doing. I need to get her indoors. I'm sorry.'

'Sorry isn't good enough, mate,' a man snapped. 'She needs to keep the hell away from our children. If you don't call the police, we will sort this out our own way.'

It was at that point that Aleena's husband decided to call the police himself, afraid for her safety and his own.

'I'm sorry, dear,' he whispered in her ear. 'I just don't know what else to do.'

As ever, the psychiatric unit was the furthest point from the hospital's car park and to reach the entrance of Nelson ward I had a long walk along a seemingly never-ending, stone-tiled corridor that smelt of iron and carbolic acid. Close your eyes and you could have been in a Victorian pharmacy.

It was summer 2013, one of the sunniest on record, and I was on the cusp of a big change. My encounter with Hayden had signalled the beginning of the end. Not just of my time at Laurel House but of my emotional threshold in dealing with the steady drip of sex offenders and system failures that flooded my in-tray and got under my skin. I'd made the decision to wind down my private practice in order to work in mainstream mental-health services exclusively with women. I had accepted a consultant psychologist post within a private group of recovery hospitals. It was the job I felt held the most promise of being able to serve a useful purpose. When the request to assess Aleena had been made by the head of psychology at the NHS hospital where she had been taken under police escort following the ugly scene in the cul-de-sac, it seemed like a fitting way to round off one era before beginning another.

Nobody came when I pressed the buzzer on the door so I peered through the slightly warped toughened safety glass. On the wall opposite was the 'Staff on Duty Today' board, centre stage of which was a photograph of a woman with her hair twisted into a high grey bun – the nurse in charge

(NIC), Roselyne. The smile on her round, scrubbed and shiny face was so infectious that I found myself twinkling back at her, only to quickly adjust my face before anyone spotted me interacting with a notice board.

I pressed the buzzer again and, after another minute or two, a hot and harassed-looking nursing assistant appeared and let me in.

'Sorry to keep you waiting, love,' she said, fanning her face with her hand. 'We're all chasing our tails, as usual.'

As we set off down the main corridor to the nurse's office, a tall man with long, straggly hair fell into step with us. He was wearing a blue T-shirt with the slogan 'Lawyers do it in their briefs' printed on it.

'Hello,' I said, giving him a nodding acknowledgement.

He stared back at me, saying nothing and, once I was installed in the empty nursing office he stood outside, still poker-faced and with his nose millimetres from the window.

Acknowledging why nursing stations are often referred to as 'the goldfish bowl', I stood up and started looking at the chart drawn on a large whiteboard on the back wall of the room. It was divided into 25 rows, one for each of the nine female patients and 16 men on this acute ward.

I located Aleena's handwritten name, her age and date of birth and followed the row to see that she was detained under Section 3 of the Mental Health Act, meaning she was hospitalized for treatment that was deemed necessary for her health, her safety or for the protection of other people. With the T-shirt guy's eyes burning into the side of my head, it felt like an age before the NIC arrived to meet me. Roselyne was as buoyant as she looked in her photograph, though that didn't last long.

'Welcome, welcome. Now remind me, which patient are you here to see?'

As soon as she heard Aleena's name it was as though a shadow fell across her face. Flaring her nostrils and pursing her lips into a tight button, she shook her head. 'I don't know what to make of that one. She's been in and out of here like a yo-yo over the past four years.' Roselyne then let out a rather despondent laugh, adding, 'She's definitely a heartsink patient.'

'Heartsink patients' are those considered time-consuming, troublesome, manipulative and difficult to help. This disparaging term was coined in GP practice but has crept into mental-health settings and beyond. The plunge of mood can run both ways, of course. I've met my fair share of 'heartsink professionals' who seem to specialize in making already hopeless people feel even more pessimistic that they will ever get their needs met. And I'd bet my mortgage that one or two of my clients have felt their heart sink to their boots during my own less glorious moments.

'You'll see,' said Roselyne as she logged me onto a computer so I could read Aleena's notes. Then she left me to it, promising to pop back later.

Navigating an alien computer system is one of my least favourite things. I'm always afraid I'll press the wrong button and delete swathes of unrecoverable history. My one-man audience had given me one last, lingering once-over before wandering off, so at least I could focus on the job in hand without feeling like an exhibit at the London Aquarium.

I'd been asked to provide a specialist assessment of Aleena's risk of violence. An unusual request from a hospital, not least in these cash-strapped times, but the head of psychology explained that the clinical psychologist attached to the psychiatric wards felt that she had neither the time nor the expertise for the task required.

'Wouldn't your local forensic service be willing to offer an opinion?' I'd asked. Sad to say, but with regular mental-health services stretched to breaking point at that time, if you wanted a half-decent assessment and a conscientious risk-management plan for someone, usually the only option was to refer them to forensic services (which was at least preferable to waiting until they seriously harmed someone and then letting the courts do it for you).

'They reviewed the paperwork but turned down the referral. That's why we have come to you. There is a lot of concern surrounding this lady's behaviour.'

Aleena's admission summary told me she was the elder of two sisters born to Iraqi-Kurdish parents living in Brighton. Her first contact with psychiatric services had been at the ripe old age of 42 but she had carouselled in and out of Nelson ward ever since, staying for up to three months at a time. She'd amassed the seemingly compulsory collection of diagnoses throughout these years, including 'schizophrenia', 'depressive disorder' and – *quelle surprise* – 'borderline personality disorder'. Her current label was 'paranoid schizophrenia', a subtype of schizophrenia where feelings or beliefs of persecution are prominent (and which, by the way, had just been taken out of the latest version of the *Big Book of Human Suffering*, along with all other subtypes of schizophrenia, due to its 'limited diagnostic stability,[1] low reliability and poor validity').

The string of shift diary entries mainly told me that Aleena was 'accepting of diet and fluids' and 'visible in communal areas'. Typical phrases that appear in notes in mental-health services across the land, despite being laughably unhelpful. The last one was there to demonstrate that Aleena was not holed up in her bedroom for the entirety of the shift but always gave me a mental image of apparitions carrying floating paper cups of medication and shouting 'boo' at the night staff.

The next page of diary entries was far more enlightening, telling me that Aleena had 'further periods of screaming loudly, for up to two hours'. The screaming was described as 'wailing at high volume, upsetting fellow patients'. Three days ago, she'd been given additional tranquillizing medication because she had been pacing up and down the ward, repeatedly stating, 'I need to see blood.'

Now I was getting somewhere.

I opened up a file marked 'Risk Assessment and Management'. Every patient in a psychiatric facility has a

---

[1]   This means that the diagnosis would often be classed as something else upon subsequent meetings with psychiatrists.

risk assessment. Although different hospitals and institutions have their own preferred tools for the job, as a minimum each must address the same three basic areas: the likelihood of self-harm and/or suicide, the possibility of the patient being exploited by anyone during their admission and any risks they might pose to the safety of others. The starting point for identifying such risks is always a thorough analysis of the individual's history, because it is both a truism and a grossly oversimplified maxim that 'the best predictor of future behaviour is past behaviour'.

Aleena's risk assessment listed numerous episodes of self-harm. The latest had taken place just a couple of days earlier and was run-of-the-mill for her, it appeared. 'She used her fingernails to scratch the top of her forehead until blood poured down her face,' it read. It struck me that the word 'poured' sounded a little dramatic. Head wounds do bleed more profusely than injuries to other parts of the body due to the high number of blood vessels in the face and scalp, but I couldn't imagine blood 'pouring' like a waterfall from wounds inflicted by fingernails. Aleena's risk in this area was what I would describe as 'high frequency, low harm'. Although she often dug her nails into her face, hands or arms until her skin tore, she had never deliberately harmed herself in a more serious or life-threatening way.

Next, I searched for her history of violent behaviour. I naturally assumed there must be some because, after all, wasn't this what I'd been drafted in to provide an expert excavation of? Curiously, aside from the fracas that had led to her admission, the risk assessment gave up nothing. Zilch, nada, not a sausage. I was still scowling in confusion at the computer screen when Roselyne returned.

'There are no other risk markers for violence, so am I missing something?' I asked. And that's when I started to get a much clearer picture of why I'd been brought in.

The NHS Trust had experienced more than its fair share of 'serious untoward incidents' over the past few years, Roselyne told me, in a voice loaded with opprobrium. Eight months previously, a male patient from Nelson ward had failed to return on time after visiting the hospital canteen. He'd eaten a shepherd's pie and plate of chips, then walked up to the second storey of the car park and jumped.

'He landed on the bonnet of a car being driven by one of the out-patients from the neurology department,' she added. 'Both of them ended up with broken bones and the neurology patient received terrible head injuries.'

'Oh blimey,' I said, blinking at the cruel irony of that last detail.

'The post-incident review team came up with a whole list of recommendations for improved practice,' Roselyne tutted, 'though most of them were totally impractical, of course. We just don't have the time or the staff numbers.'

So I was one of the practical recommendations, was I? Hired to help meet a directive that the hospital was now required to implement? Now I get it, I thought. I wasn't only there to tick boxes. I *was* a ticked box.

Roselyne must have seen the sceptical look in my eyes. She

took the computer mouse and swiftly scrolled down to the 'any other risk behaviour' section at the bottom of Aleena's form.

'This will make things clearer,' she said.

I read the entry out loud: 'Aleena makes comments indicating that she wants to harm people, specifically female children.'

Before I could say any more, Roselyne was quick to jump in, explaining that Aleena had a habit of repeating 'I want to see blood' or 'I want to see the blood of little girls.'

'Worrying, isn't it?' she asked, but didn't wait for an answer. 'We are *extremely* worried that she might carry out her threats. She is very ill. And she is currently on a large combination of medication but it hasn't touched the sides, I'm afraid. She is still as mad as a box of frogs.'

'We're all mad here,' I said, quoting *Alice in Wonderland,* because I had long ago rejected the notion that there is a separate group of people who are 'mentally ill'. There are just some who encounter more extreme distress than others as we all try our best to survive what life has thrown at us.

Roselyne looked blankly at me.

'What else can you tell me?' I asked.

'Where do I start? When she was first admitted, Aleena put blobs of her own blood on the foreheads of the female staff and patients, blood she'd scratched out of her own forehead. Then she tried to draw on all the women's hands on the ward with a red marker pen, causing mayhem. And, about two weeks ago, there was the debacle in the art-therapy class.'

'What happened there?'

311

'She poured a bottle of red paint all over herself and the walls. She also smeared paint all over the therapist's hands. At that point, we took the decision to stop her from attending any more art-therapy classes. The next time she might draw her own or someone else's blood with the end of a paintbrush or some other implement. It is simply too big a risk to take.'

It struck me as a strange overreaction but I chose my words carefully. 'It sounds to me like she only quite literally *draws* blood on other people,' I offered.

Roselyne looked at me as though she didn't understand but she didn't ask me to clarify what I meant. 'If she hurt someone, even after discharge – and especially if it was a child – the unit could be closed down. Beds are being cut all across the hospital. One more cock-up and they won't have to look too far to decide which unit is next.'

'I'm sure it won't come to that,' I replied, in what I hoped was my most zen-like voice, the one I use in relaxation sessions with my patients. 'I plan to do as thorough an assessment as possible.'

Roselyne seemed placated. She had helped me enormously to understand the psychological make-up of my client. Or one of them at least. When you agree to work with any individual as a forensic psychologist, you also take on the people and institutions who hold the keys, both literal and figurative, to the doors that confine them. I now understood all too well the collective psyche of the hospital staff who had hired me. Aleena, meanwhile, was still a conundrum.

*

A nursing assistant, whose badge said James but who insisted everyone called him Jimbo, walked me down the corridor to the communal lounge area, which was a soulless rectangular space lined with rows of armchairs covered in flame-retardant, phlegm-green fabric. A television was positioned high on the wall and several patients were sitting around dozing off or watching house hunters being shown around a chateau in the Dordogne.

'There she is, with the black hair,' Jimbo signalled to me.

I could see Aleena in profile, her face pointed at the screen and a glossy braid of hair falling halfway down her back.

I'd spent an hour making telephone calls chasing Aleena's previous admission and community-team notes. I had also managed a short conversation with her consultant psychiatrist. I'd discovered that she'd been working at a primary school five years ago, until one day when she was found hiding in the classroom cupboard. Complaints had already been received from parents and guardians who had noticed that their girls were arriving home every day with circles of red felt-tip pen and paint on their hands and face. Aleena explained to her head teacher that disembodied 'eyeballs' were following her, saying she had seen them peeking over her garden fence at home and peering into windows. Once she had been coaxed out of the cupboard, she was encouraged to visit her GP and hadn't returned to her post since.

Aleena was made a psychiatric in-patient for the first time after her community mental-health nurse visited her at home and found her smeared with her own blood. She was talking too rapidly and incoherently to be understood. Her husband, Jason, was finding it difficult to cope and told the nurse that Aleena was barely leaving the house by herself anymore. When she did, she had started stopping neighbours and scaring them with talk of 'the eyes'.

Aleena hadn't resisted being admitted to Nelson ward, but her bouts of shrieking and preoccupation with blood made her an intimidating and unpopular presence among fellow patients. She had 'failed to develop any insight into her illness', her psychiatrist told me, but she nevertheless passively accepted the medication she was prescribed until she eventually 'settled down' and was discharged. (*If she was compliant, did she even need to be detained under the Mental Health Act?* I wondered.) She had repeated this pattern six times over the last four years.

I could see that Aleena was placid now. She looked like she was gazing at her own reflection in the TV screen rather than watching the presenter unveil the kidney-shaped swimming pool. The man in the T-shirt was there too, appearing far more interested in Aleena than in the property show.

Aleena turned towards us when she heard our footsteps. She was a very handsome woman with big, expressive eyes and enviably thick eyelashes. She was striking for another reason too – blood was dribbling in thin lines down her face, like tiny rivulets of rain on a window pane.

'Hello, Aleena, I'm Kerry. Can I have a chat with you?'

I put my hand out, just in time to see that some blood had transferred to her hands. It wasn't ideal, but so what? I've touched a lot worse and I was up to date with all my jabs, hepatitis included.

Aleena didn't take my hand but she did say hello and nodded her head as she got to her feet. She was a short woman with solid legs clad in navy-blue shorts. Standing square to me, she touched her temples, dabbing at some of the lines of blood running from what looked like old wounds she had opened up on her forehead.

'We can go to the visitors' room,' I told her, hoping we would have some privacy there.

Without saying a word Aleena reached for my face, stroking my cheek gently with her bloodied fingertips. It was a novel greeting and my first thought was that I must have looked like a hunter smeared with their first kill.

'Shall we go?' I asked, gesturing down the pale green corridor.

But before we had a chance to take more than a step, we were intercepted by Roselyne, who came barrelling towards us in a cloud of faux outrage.

'What have you done to this nice lady?' she demanded. 'She's a *psychologist*! This is not acceptable, Aleena.'

'It's alright,' I started, but Jimbo had reappeared in Roselyne's wake and was already ushering Aleena out of the lounge. T-shirt man was getting out of his seat, seemingly in two minds whether or not to follow.

I watched, dumbfounded, as my client was whisked away from me. Roselyne had pulled out a tissue from her pocket and was churning the saliva in her mouth so audibly that, for one horrifying moment, I thought that she was about to spit on it and wipe my face with it, like my grandmother used to do when I was a child.

'Honestly, it's fine. I'm fine with it,' I said, recoiling. 'As bodily fluids at work go, blood is absolutely my favourite.'

She put an unnecessary arm around me and swept me back into the nursing office where she swabbed me down with a wet wipe, apologizing profusely as she scrubbed at my cheek until it was as spotless and rosy as her own. By the time she'd finished, I wasn't sure whether I was thoroughly irritated or begrudgingly endeared by her. I decided it was both. I didn't have much choice now but to abandon my plan to start working with Aleena that afternoon. She was nowhere to be seen as I was escorted to the ward entrance to begin the trek back to my car.

As we reached the 'Staff on Duty Today' photographs, I was hit by a raw and piercing scream. It sounded like a wounded animal. It seemed to slice straight through the warm afternoon air, turning it ice cold. I shivered, the hairs on my arms prickling my skin like tiny frozen needles.

The next morning, Aleena was brought to the visitors' room to see me, where I was optimistic that we'd finally be able to talk without interruption. She looked overly sedated, her dark eyes half-closed and unreadable, and she rolled her neck from side to side as though she had been sleeping for a long time at an awkward angle.

I explained the reason why I had been asked to see her.

'We did risk assessments at the school where I worked,' she stated, her voice sounding deep and drowsy. 'Why do I need to be risk assessed?'

The first response that came to mind was: *Because the hospital psychiatry services are feeling under threat and have employed my services as an arse-covering exercise.* Tempting, but I opted instead to give the more official answer.

'Every patient on the ward is risk assessed. But I've been asked to help out with your assessment because people have been worried by the way you behaved with your neighbours' children a few weeks ago. And by some of the things that you say. So, I want to try and understand you better and make sure you get the right help.'

She bobbed her head lightly in assent.

I was carrying out an HCR-20 assessment, I told her, showing her the blue and orange booklet where I was making my notes. HCR stands for Historical, Clinical, Risk Management and is a tool that prompts you to think about the presence and relevance of 20 factors, each proposed to be associated with the risk of future violence in 'mentally disordered' people. The HCR-20 is a huge piece of work, guiding you, as it does, through a series of steps in order to make an educated guess about what kind of violence a person may perpetrate, against whom, for which reasons and under what circumstances. The end goal is to prevent any predicted violence by developing plans for future intervention.

I use the term 'educated guess' advisedly because all types of violence risk assessment have limitations. Structured approaches like the HCR-20 work better than relying on a psychologist's individual judgement alone (which is about as error-free as casting some rune stones). But still, they don't grant you any Nostradamus-like powers of prophecy and it is simply impossible to foretell the future with anything close to full accuracy.

Not only that, but research shows that when it comes to foreseeing *rare* forms of violence (such as a 46-year-old woman with no previous history of instability or antisocial behaviour harming an unrelated child), any kind of risk assessment is poor and will produce far more false-positive predictions of violence than true ones.

Those realities aside, I'd promised Roselyne I'd do a thorough job, worthy of the mistress of doom herself, and that is what I intended to do. Besides, I was itching to hear what Aleena had to say. I wanted to unpick her motivations for covering herself and other females in red marks, and I wanted to figure out whether her desire to 'see blood' was, in fact, evidence of violent ideas – as everyone around her seemed to have already decided was the case – or something else entirely. But all in good time. First, I planned to talk through aspects of Aleena's general history as a subtle lead into the more confronting questions I'd ask later.

It was a slow conversation but I wasn't in a rush.

'My husband is a kind man, a very kind man,' Aleena yawned as she started telling me about the important people in her life. 'He is my one and only.'

'Is it just the two of you at home?'

'We had a dog, my dog. He was an Akita, called Prince. He died a few months ago.'

I said I was sorry, telling her I was a dog lover and knew the Japanese breed.

'They're loyal and noble, aren't they? What was Prince like?' I asked.

'He was always by my side. I miss him so much. Not long after he died, I lost my nurse too.'

She was referring to her community mental-health nurse, an almost weekly visitor to her home for over two years until she had retired.

'They sent me a new nurse. I didn't let him in.'

'Why not?' I asked.

Aleena didn't answer, she seemed distracted and then suddenly froze.

The guy in the T-shirt had appeared in the glass viewing panel in the door. He had been there on and off for most of the time that Aleena and I had been talking, being intermittently shooed away by one of the nursing assistants.

'We are being watched,' Aleena whispered, leaning forwards.

'By who?'

I instinctively glanced at our deadpan spectator, though I realized she was not referring to him.

'The eyes. The eyes are in the room.'

'I can't see them, Aleena. Where are they?'

She pointed to the water dispenser at the back of the room, empty and littered with clear plastic cups.

'Do you know who the eyes belong to?'

She nodded and started to breathe heavily, digging her fingernails tightly into the back of her left hand, which was already covered with raised scars and claret-coloured scabs of skin. Out of nowhere, a thunderous banging sound made us both jump in our seats. Our uninvited observer had chosen that moment to kick the bottom of the door before walking off.

Aleena stopped clawing at her hand and looked at me in shock.

'That wasn't helpful of him, was it?' I said. 'Are you alright?'

'Blue eyes, brown eyes,' she panted. 'Have they brought shame on you?'

It was a question to the room, not to me.

'Mothers let them watch their babies, mothers let them watch their babies,' she repeated.

'I don't understand, Aleena.'

She repeated it again and again, her impassioned and despairing words escaping like pressure from a punctured aerosol can. There was a message in there but, frustratingly for us both, I couldn't make sense of it.

Aleena's stare was fixed on me now and she gave a little squeak. Her mouth fell open and she looked skywards, her eyes rolling upwards in her head until only the whites of them were visible.

Shit, I thought, *she's having an oculogyric crisis!* I had only seen it a handful of times before. It's where the muscles that control the eyes go into spasm. It can be painful and it's a severe side-effect of antipsychotic medication, although fatigue and stress will also help it along.

Aleena was scraping hard at her hand. I took it as lightly as possible in my own.

'Aleena, Aleena. I think that you are having a side-effect to the medication you are taking. It's going to be alright. I'm just going to get a nurse to help you.'

I headed to the door and waved wildly at the nearest member of staff. Five minutes later, Aleena was being attended to by Roselyne and an on-call doctor. I decided to give them some space and made my way to the lounge area. As I dropped down onto a rubbery armchair, a long sigh of air escaped from it. *You as well? That's just how I feel,* I thought. If I were in Aleena's shoes, being pursued by nefarious body parts, the last place I would want to be was in here, locked up with T-shirt man and where the only 'treatment' on offer was being drugged up to the literal eyeballs.

And they call this a therapeutic environment!

I was suddenly beginning to second-guess my decision to go back to hospital work. And, more pressingly, whether I'd ever get to have a full conversation with my client.

At least I could talk to Aleena's husband. Jason visited every other day and, with her agreement, I'd arranged to speak to him that afternoon. I'd expected he'd help fill in some of the many gaps in my assessment but he did more besides.

Jason was an unassuming man with a low, gravelly voice. 'I just want my wife back,' he told me. 'I love her, but some days I don't recognize her.'

They had met in college when they were both teenagers. 'Aleena was keen to get away from home because her parents were very strict, very traditional. They weren't pleased with her for having a relationship with a white man but she was a free spirit. She wanted to live up north after finishing her studies so she ended up moving in with me and my mother in Cheshire. After that, I guess she never had much contact with her own family. They are a long way away, still living down on the south coast, where she grew up.'

Aleena married Jason – now an electrical engineer – as soon as she'd finished her teacher training. They continued living with his mother until she passed away several years later. It meant Aleena and Jason were both approaching 30 by the time they moved to their current home, at the top of the cul-de-sac in one of Manchester's most genteel suburbs.

'It's a cliché but we had it all. A lovely detached house, no money worries. Before Aleena got ill she was in a running club. She loved that, and we were always cycling together, whenever we could. In the school holidays I took time off and we travelled around Europe in our camper van.'

'Did you notice any problems at all with her emotional state?'

'I'd say she's always been a worrier,' he replied. 'She over-thinks things but she never had mental problems, not until...'

At this point, small patches of perspiration started to appear under his arm. He told me her problems seemed to start after she turned 40. 'She, um, hit the, you know, the menopause very early, you see,' he stuttered.

He loosened a button on the top of his shirt and I wondered if he was squeamish about 'women's problems'. That type of prudishness always leaves me battling the urge to say the word 'vagina' as many times and as loudly as I can, just to enjoy the reaction. But that wasn't it.

He gave a nervous cough. 'Can I tell you something?'

'Yes, of course you can. Please do.'

'But I don't want it written down. I don't want Aleena to know.'

I gave him my well-rehearsed little speech, the one about not being able to keep information confidential that might put himself or anyone else at risk. I cringed as I recited it, knowing I sounded like a robot and telling myself I had to work a bit harder on my delivery.

'Oh, right.' Jason said, looking torn. 'Maybe I shouldn't. Although I don't think it puts anyone at risk.'

I put my pen down and looked at him across the coffee table that sat between us, showing him I was ready and willing to listen.

'The thing is,' he said, so softly I was straining to hear him, 'me and Aleena had always envisaged having children one day. We argued about it at times, about when we should do it. Now, full disclosure here...' He stopped talking and looked up to the ceiling for a moment. 'We agreed to just see if it happened, but I started to... change my mind. I liked our lifestyle and I didn't want it to change. We'd had years of living with my mother. I liked it just being the two of us, being able to take off on our bikes or on holiday whenever we wanted...'

He dropped his head forward, staring at his trainers as if they were a fascinating work of art.

'The thing is, I had a vasectomy. She doesn't know.'

It's amazing the secrets you get to hear in this job, I thought. I could see why Jason would want to tie heavy weights around that one and leave it to sleep with the fishes. Rather than face a difficult conversation, he'd taken matters into his own hands, denying Aleena the chance to make an informed decision of whether to stay with him or pursue her dreams of a family elsewhere. It was quite an admission but it was not for me to reproach him.

'Right,' I said quietly. 'I understand.'

Jason had not finished yet. Stealing a glance at me, he admitted he was privately relieved when his wife began the menopause early. *I bet you were*, I thought. But instead of it drawing a line under her hopes of having children, the menopause brought Aleena no peace at all, he explained.

'In fact, the opposite was true,' he frowned. 'Because that's when she started acting weird. I'd find her hiding in the pantry or locked in the bathroom. And she only left the house if she was going to work, or cycling or running, and only then if Prince was with her.'

Jason was scratching the top of his head with both hands, looking defeated and perplexed.

'Did you talk to her about it?' I asked, sensing that I already knew the answer.

'I just told her there was nothing to worry about, there was nobody watching her or following her. I thought she was just depressed or something, you know, because she'd had to accept that we weren't going to have children. I thought it would get better, but then the doctor said she had schizophrenia.'

'How did you feel about that?'

'Guilty. Frightened. I'd find her covered with blood. One day she poured a bottle of tomato ketchup over herself. When I cleaned her up she screamed the house down. And this latest thing with the neighbours was terrible. I'm scared of what she will do next.'

'Has she ever threatened to harm anybody?' I asked gently.

'No.'

'Has she ever told you that she has thoughts of harming anybody?'

'No, not really. She just keeps on saying she wants to see blood. I tell her all the time not to say it but she gets obsessed.'

'Has she ever been violent towards you, or anybody else that you know of?'

'Never, Aleena's not normally a violent person. She absolutely loved the kids she worked with, she would do anything for them, and she was always gentle with Prince. I've never felt scared of her. But I suppose anything is possible because she is ill. Her menopause seems to have triggered this awful mental disease.'

It struck me how unquestioningly people separate what they accept are symptoms of 'mental disease' from any valid motivation on the part of the person concerned, as though they have been robbed of their humanity and are incapable of any rational thought at all. Jason had shared his life with Aleena for almost 30 years and yet, as he said himself, he could hardly recognize her anymore. All he could see was plain 'schizophrenia', an illness that rendered her unpredictable and potentially dangerous, rather than behaviours that were shaped by and intertwined with the very essence of who she was.

It was at that moment that I decided that it was time for me to immerse myself in Aleena's world, blood and all. Aleena badly needed somebody willing to walk in the 'madness' alongside her without fear, open to listening and looking for the meaning within it.

It took me a whole day and several conversations – not just with the head of psychology but with Aleena's psychiatrist and the ward manager – to be granted permission to use the art room for three hours.

Knowing how risk-averse the whole hospital trust was, I had my health-and-safety hat on when I put in my request, asking for a small pack of non-toxic ready-mixed paints (the sort that washes out and doesn't poison children even if they decide to drink it), some plain sheets of paper and the use of a couple of their largest, blunt and extremely non-lethal paintbrushes. I also agreed in writing that I wouldn't claim expenses if Aleena doused me in paint and said I'd clear up any mess if she chucked it up the walls again.

Aleena seemed tense as we sat in the art room. To me, it smelled friendly, like plasticine and children's parties. But her eyes flitted past the luminous watercolour landscapes, charcoal portraits and papier maché hot-air balloons on display. She was searching the windows, I realized. Was she checking to see if anyone – or perhaps anything – was keeping an eye on us?

I speedily sellotaped six sheets of A2 paper together and invited her to do some painting, if she wanted to. After a minute or two, she selected the little bottle of red paint and began to squeeze it all over our makeshift canvas. Then she picked up a paintbrush, dabbed it in the paint and started swirling it in slow circles. The effect was immediate. Seeing the swathes of red appearing on the white paper seemed to have a calmative effect, the tightness around her jaw softening and her initially stiff body starting to sway naturally with the rhythm of her brush strokes.

I picked up a paintbrush too and started twirling it in the paint, and silently and together we filled more of the paper in garish, letter-box red.

Aleena sat backwards and put her head to one side to fully take in our artwork and then she splodged big blobs of paint straight from the bottle on to the palms of each of her hands. As a former Catholic schoolgirl, I was reminded of stigmata. With the network of scars and healing scrapes laced across her forehead, Aleena made me think of those statues of Jesus, blood on his outstretched hands and with the crown of thorns on his head.

Without saying a word, she then held her paintbrush out towards me. I held my hands out, imagining she wanted to put paint on the middle of my palms too, which was fine by me. Except that wasn't her intention at all. Aleena instead reached across and daubed a massive dot of red paint on my forehead, right between my eyes. It took me so much by surprise that I had to laugh. I was even more surprised when Aleena let out a short, ringing burst of the giggles too.

'I must look a right sight,' I commented.

'It's good, it's paint-blood, blood-paint!' she smiled, returning to the canvas, making wavy lines and swirls as she swept her brush through the paint.

'I don't mind,' I told her. 'But not everybody appreciates you putting paint-blood on them. In fact, some people get pretty frightened by it, you know.'

'I *want* to see blood,' she said. She was petulant in her tone. 'Mothers don't care about their babies,' she went on. 'They let them watch their babies, they don't care.'

'You haven't told me much about your own parents yet. Did your mother do a good job of caring for you?'

I saw Aleena's grip tighten around her paintbrush and the curves and waves she was painting flattened into harder, straighter lines. Her mouth pulled sideways and set into a defiant line.

'My mother was perfect on the outside but a weak woman on the inside,' she announced, while blinking rapidly.

'What makes you feel that?'

There was a momentary pause. Aleena lowered the paintbrush, splaying the bristles haphazardly on the paper. She joined her hands together, watching the red paint ooze through her fingers before streaking it over her fists. Then she proceeded to tell me, a little disjointedly, that she had been sexually assaulted and raped as a child. It happened on multiple occasions from the age of seven, by a group of three attackers, her two 18-year-old neighbours and one of their friends.

'They would spy over the garden fence at me and follow me when I was sent to run errands or buy milk and dolma from the corner shop. They took me back to their house or put me in their car. They said that I must enjoy it. But if I ever told anyone, they would do it to my baby sister instead.'

'I'm so sorry you were subjected to that. Did you ever feel able to tell someone?'

Aleena nodded. 'When I was ten years old. My sister had just had her seventh birthday. And she slapped me.'

'Slapped you?' I repeated. 'Your sister?'

'My perfect mother, she slapped me. It was the only time in my life she ever hit me. She said I had brought dishonour on the whole family and she made me promise never to speak of it. Never let my father hear of it, or anyone else. She said that if I did, no respectable Kurdish husband would want to match with me and the whole family would be disgraced.'

She wiped a hand across her cheek, inadvertently smearing herself with a stripe of colour as she did so.

'When did it end, Aleena?'

'When I was 12. When I started to bleed.'

'Do you mean when you started your periods?'

Aleena held her hands up triumphantly before lowering her voice as much as possible, as though she had a great wisdom to share with me. 'They hate blood. It disgusts them. It drives them away.' She was laughing now.

Of course it drove them away, I thought to myself. *You had reached puberty, and had you fallen pregnant, they would have risked being exposed.*

Aleena had straightened her spine and lifted her chin up. She had shared her hard-won knowledge and seemed delighted with it but she was keen to move on, and fast. I went with her.

'Please, please don't tell my husband,' she implored me. 'You cannot tell him. I have never told him any of this. I don't want him to think badly of me.'

I promised her that I wouldn't, but I also told her she had nothing at all to be ashamed of. The bitterness Aleena expressed towards her mother suggested that she knew that, but often knowing something intellectually is quite different from being able to fully absorb it emotionally.

I've encountered numerous victims of sexual abuse who have not been believed when they've finally plucked up the courage to disclose their abuse to family or friends, whether as children or as adults. It is almost harder to comprehend, but every bit as common, when they *are* believed, yet blamed for their own abuse. What a double-whammy of betrayal that is, being told by someone you have confided in that you are somehow responsible for one of the most psychologically ruinous things that can be inflicted on a person.

I sometimes ask victims and survivors of sexual violence (my 'warriors', if that is what they choose to call themselves) to imagine their abuser or abusers wearing a bulky overcoat. The coat belongs to them and has deep pockets filled with the guilt, shame and responsibility for the abuse they have carried out. It is heavy and threatens to swamp them, no longer allowing them to continue to justify to themselves what it is they want to do. So they take it off and instead they hang it on their victim. Too often, when others hear of the abuse, rather than helping the victim to unpack the pockets and to shrug off a burden that was never theirs in the first place, fear and ignorance compel them to sew another pocket of blame into the coat and fill it with their own misguided beliefs about how the victim might have invited or failed to properly resist the assault.

Aleena's mother had done just that, convinced she had to ensure her daughter's future silence at all costs. Her reaction didn't just serve to quiet Aleena on the matter, it caused her young daughter to internalize the belief that she had contravened the moral code a female of her background must adhere to in order to remain valuable. In other words, the coat, and all it carried, was somehow hers.

How frightening it must have been to ask the most trusted person in her world for help, only to realize that none was available. Speaking up had only served to create more humiliation and fear, a burden that must have been so confusing for a ten-year-old girl to carry alone. It was obvious how and why blood – or anything symbolizing blood – was significant to Aleena. The onset of her menstrual bleeds had been the only thing she had learned would protect her.

*

The paint on my face had dried into a tight, itchy crust by the time Roselyne had me practically pinned to the wall in the nurse's office, chipping it off.

'There you go,' she said with satisfaction, 'you just look a little sunburned. I'd better go and see if Lady Macbeth is all cleaned up too.'

It looked like my love–hate relationship with the nurse in charge was set to continue.

'But she was guilty of murder,' I retorted.

'What?'

'Lady Macbeth. She murdered someone and then hallucinated blood on her hands. It's not the same as Aleena.'

'Oh. Well, anyway, I'll go and see if she needs a wipe over. I can't leave her covered in paint.'

'Why not?' *Let her bathe in the stuff if it makes her feel less threatened,* I thought.

I confess that I had expected to end the day scouring paint off the walls and ceiling but, when I raised no objection to Aleena giving herself (and my forehead) a coat or two of paint, her behaviour hadn't escalated into anything problematic. We had left the art room just as we had found it and, though I might have resembled a red-headed woodpecker, I'd clearly managed, with no trouble at all, to avoid assault by paintbrush.

Roselyne had armed herself with a fresh packet of wet wipes, ready to tackle Aleena. 'We can't have patients running about head-to-toe in paint, it isn't right.'

'Oh, it's mostly her hands,' I cajoled. 'And perhaps it *is* right, for her at the moment. Couldn't you let her choose to wash it off when she wants?'

Roselyne narrowed her eyes. 'I suppose it can't do any harm.'

'Thank you, you are a gem.'

I was feeling upbeat as I emptied a king's ransom in small change into the parking machine at the end of the day. Walking away from the unit, I'd been mulling over how easy it had been to get to the nub of Aleena's behaviour.

But then I couldn't help wondering why these conversations hadn't taken place in the four years that she had been yo-yoing in and out of hospital.

I'd assumed Aleena had been asked similar questions before but had simply never given an answer. Maybe the setting was wrong or perhaps her frame of mind at the time prevented her from answering? I didn't know, but there were no records of any such conversations. There had been ward rounds and Care Programme Approach (CPA) meetings, where Aleena would sit surrounded by professionals to be told what 'illness' she had and what medication she would be prescribed to eradicate her 'symptoms'. There had been conversations with doctors and nurses – and with her husband, as he had described – about how she mustn't scratch holes in her skin, mustn't cover herself or others in red substances and would she please stop talking about blood and stop screaming?

When people scream, they scream for a reason.

So much time and money had been fed into Aleena's care and yet seemingly with so little attempt to discover what had happened in her life and what sense she had made of it. What thought had been given to how her past might be shaping the way she was experiencing and expressing her pain? I found it both depressingly typical and utterly astonishing. As Professor of Psychiatry Joel Gold and his brother Ian Gold wrote in *Suspicious Minds: How Culture Shapes Madness,* 'When we listen closely to what our patients are saying, paying attention to psychotic and non-psychotic thought with equal consideration, we foster the therapeutic alliance, and stronger alliances yield better therapeutic outcomes. The fact that delusions [and hallucinations] mean something to our patients is reason enough for them to mean something to us.'

Driving home, I thought back over everything that had happened in the art room that day. As we had been busy turning our sheets of paper from white to red, Aleena had told me that she had spent years watching over her sister, not letting her leave the house alone if she could help it. She didn't mind, she said, and she loved her company. She only wished that she saw more of her now they were adults.

When she told me that she had always hoped to have children I had felt my heart contract a little. She said that when it didn't happen, she felt ashamed. 'I had fallen short in my role as a wife. I wondered if I was of less value to my husband.' She allowed herself a half smile. 'Silly thoughts,' she said, explaining that they were firmly rooted in the conservative Kurdish values she grew up with.

I gritted my teeth and said nothing of Jason's secret; it was not mine to reveal and could only serve to hurt her further now.

As a teenager and young woman, Aleena had always felt 'joy' and 'relief' when her period came because to her the blood represented safety. As time went on, her failure to conceive (as she saw it) caused her relationship with her own body to become more complicated. A roller-coaster of hope, anticipation and disappointment every month. Then, when she approached the menopause, her periods arriving less and less frequently as she reached the end of her thirties, a familiar surge of abject betrayal crashed in.

'It wasn't fair that I would never have children. I would have been a good mother, dedicated to my family. I thought about it for a long time. My own body had let me down, that's how it felt, that's what had happened.'

It was within this commotion of physical and emotional upheaval and uncertainty that Aleena started to hallucinate. 'Blue eyes, brown eyes, staring at me through the window. Blue eyes, brown eyes, looking into my classroom at work.'

I wondered if Aleena was seeing the menacing eyes of her childhood rapists, eyes that had only stopped tracking her when she had reached puberty. But the mind rarely takes such clear-cut routes.

'Who do the eyes belong to, do you think?'

'They are windows to the soul, the souls of sly men, immoral men. They send them to spy on me.' She was searching my face now, checking to see if I believed her. 'They tell me I'm crazy but I *know* it's true. I see them, I've seen them looking at you, too.'

When Aleena's periods stopped altogether, at the age of 42,

all hope of a baby was extinguished and, with it, I imagined, any sense of having a safety net from the attentions of any 'immoral men' who might seek to harm her.

'You must be so frightened. I know I would feel petrified if I saw eyes following me,' I told her. 'Does it help you to see blood on yourself when they are about?'

Aleena nodded, putting her brush down and placing both hands, fingers splayed and palms down, on the wet paper.

'Why do you put blood and paint-blood on other women and girls?' I asked.

Aleena looked at me and screwed up her nose as if I was querying something that was entirely self-explanatory. By that point in our conversation, I'd have said it was, but yet I was obliged to ask.

'To do what weak mothers won't, to protect them. Blood to drive the eyes away.'

Ten days later, I attended Aleena's latest Care Programme Approach meeting. It's an opportunity for everyone involved in a patient's care to get together to review how things are going, agree what is needed next and plan for how this will be achieved. As is the case with most CPA meetings in psychiatric settings, Aleena would only be invited in for the last ten minutes, after the ins and outs of her future had already been decided.

The meeting wasn't being held on Nelson ward. Acting on a recommendation in my report, Aleena had been transferred to a female-only ward, where hopefully she would gain some relief, if not from 'the eyes' then at least from the gaze of the T-shirt guy. As I passed the 'Staff on Duty Today' board as I was led through the ward, I admit I felt a little disappointed that Roselyne's picture wasn't beaming at me.

The meeting was so well attended that it had to be held in the patients' TV lounge. Aleena's psychiatrist was chairing, flanked by nurses and ward managers on one side and the head of psychology and ward psychologist on the other. In addition to Aleena's care coordinator, there were also visitors from her community team, including her freshly appointed mental-health nurse. They were all busy flicking through my risk-assessment report as I found myself a seat.

My mouth started to feel dry. Sometimes on these occasions, when your conclusions don't match with popular opinion, you find yourself about as welcome as a slug in a sandwich. Wondering what sort of reception I was about to receive was starting to make the crowded room feel airless.

I had come to the (pretty easy) conclusion that Aleena represented a low risk of violence. Granted, her behaviour was often not ideal, it had plenty of potential to alarm those around her, but – as far as anyone could predict – it was unlikely to escalate into anything dangerous. Apart from her recent history of psychosis, she did not demonstrate any evidence of the factors in the HCR-20 that are the most reliably associated with future violent offending.

In fact, I was far more concerned that Aleena might become the victim of something untoward. Those with serious mental-health difficulties are up to 14 times more likely to be subjected to a violent assault than to be arrested for one. If I was ever going to read about Aleena in my local newspaper, the most likely scenario would be that her attempts to 'protect' the women and girls in her neighbourhood had met with more disapproval than just a dry-cleaning bill.

When it came time for the meeting to discuss my report, I braced myself for the questions to come thick and fast. The pairing of 'schizophrenia' and dangerousness in the minds of even mental-health professionals is a stubbornly strong one. And no doubt one or two in the room (or maybe three or four) were also weighing up the cost that accepting my opinion might pose to their future job security, should something go awry.

But the onslaught I'd imagined never came.

I'd like to believe that my work was so meticulous that it left no room for a heated debate. Far more plausible was that we all recognized a part of Aleena's story in ourselves that day. When faced with something unknown and potentially threatening, it is natural, even somewhat helpful, to become hyper-sensitive to danger. Our minds rush to fill in the gaps in what we know and don't know in an effort to keep us safe, sometimes seeing and reacting strongly to perils that aren't really there.

Simply by asking about and listening carefully to what had happened to Aleena, and relaying it faithfully to others, it seemed that I had unlocked some shared understanding of her, and possibly even some doors.

Aleena's community mental-health team notes had shown quite clearly that her most distressed behaviours were preceded by her talking about things that increased her sense of vulnerability – the loss of Prince, her pet and protector, staff changes and even crime stories, such as the murder of Joanna Yeates, which had dominated the news at the beginning of 2011. Real, anxiety-producing events that can't be easily medicated away. Having demystified Aleena's so-called 'abnormal' reaction to these, the next obvious question was, 'What does she need to help her?' Everyone at the CPA agreed that Aleena's future care must first and foremost centre on enabling her to feel safe.

She felt most secure at home and I was keen that that was where she should return, as soon as possible. A copy of my report, carefully edited to remove the details of Aleena's childhood abuse, had been prepared for her husband. It maintained her confidentiality, just as I'd promised, but said enough to help him grasp that his wife's behaviour was not so incomprehensible, or something to be feared. The ward psychologist would meet with Jason to go through it with him and discuss ways he could better support Aleena, including not trying to prevent her from minor self-harm or trying to 'clean her up'.

She would also meet with Aleena for a few sessions to agree some short-term harmless ways that Aleena could feel confident in her ability to 'drive away the eyes', even if they involved red paint and might seem strange to onlookers. She would then refer her to the out-reach psychology service, who would allocate a therapist to continue to walk alongside Aleena in what I hoped would be a journey of understanding and healing.

Psychotherapist and activist Jo Watson argues that, in our mental-health services, 'Many stories are going unheard, unacknowledged and inevitably lost forever...the "illness" becomes the story.' Aleena might have easily become one of those, her truth lost in a psychiatric system that frequently gets it wrong. It would take many more conversations for her to feel heard, validated and safe, the building blocks for trauma recovery, but the CPA meeting felt like a beginning, at least.

Walking out of the hospital for the final time felt like a bright new beginning for me, too. I was ready to take the bold step of shutting down my private practice and starting my consultant-psychologist role, working with women in-patients, just like Aleena. If I could be a safe witness and ally to them as they pieced together their own, hidden stories, that would be valuable.

The timing felt right. I wasn't entirely sure what I was letting myself in for, but I knew I didn't feel afraid of it.

EPILOGUE

A solicitor I once worked with made the schoolboy error of giving my mobile number to our mutual client, who was running late for her appointment. She had beaten her neighbours' three-year-old child while babysitting, claiming a vague and unsubstantiated mental 'illness' in her defence. When she failed to win the result she hoped for in court, she decided that I was responsible. Now, whenever she gets a new telephone number (which seems to be every few months), I get a flurry of 3am text messages telling me – in capitals and creative detail – exactly where to shove my psychological opinion.

Her troubles are, of course, the result of her own unacceptable behaviour. But she doesn't want to examine that too closely or consider the dim view that members of the jury (whose numbers I'm guessing she hasn't got written down) formed of her, based on the evidence. Instead, she focuses her searchlight on me, time and time again, because it is more agreeable and convenient to accept my involvement as a good enough single explanation for the outcome of her trial. And perception, as the saying goes, is everything.

The popular perception is that 'madness' or 'badness' are the only two, distinct and mutually exclusive, explanations for criminal or difficult-to-tolerate behaviours. The idea has a long history and has been taken up and cultivated by modern-day media representations of the people I have spent over

25 years working with. People whose stories I have done my best to hear with a curious, compassionate and open mind – albeit with varying degrees of success – and whom I frequently fail to recognize in the portrayals that are served up daily, whether in news or fictional form, for our entertainment and information.

In many respects, I believe we have created a new Bedlam. The 'true crime' genre has become the modern-day equivalent of visiting the asylum, giving the supposedly 'sane' and 'good' among us the chance to peer through a dirty window at a world we hope only to visit and never inhabit. A world where those with mental-health problems are stigmatized for our edification. To add insult to psychological injury, those bestowed with the least understood mental-health diagnoses, or those who manifest their distress or differences in ways that we find the most uncomfortable or difficult to deal with, such as people like Aleena, are the most castigated of all.

It is rarely facts but rather our socially constructed and stereotypical notions of people, unreliable and unscientific diagnostic systems, the imposition of our own set of values about how others 'ought' to behave and illogical fears that determine who is assigned a 'mad' or 'bad' label. Labels that not only fail to reveal all the plot lines and turning points in an individual's life story but could well bury their truth forever.

My reason for writing this book is, first and foremost, to introduce you to a cross-section of the people I spend my average working week with, so you can meet them as the diverse bunch of human beings that they are. I'm also hoping that after reading about Nigel, Michael, Justine, Isaaq et al, you might feel better equipped to dig a little deeper next time you are confronted with a lazy 'mad or bad' narrative.

When I say this, I don't want to excuse poor behaviour. Embracing the complexity of people – acknowledging how we are shaped by history, our life events, relationships and circumstances, the social and cultural standards we are expected to live up to, and the extent to which we are exposed to abuse, adversity and inequality – doesn't change what is right and what is wrong. Any behaviour that harms others or breaks the shared rules of our society is unacceptable. However, when we view people in their full context, we find that many forms of disturbed and disturbing behaviour become understandable, at least. And we learn that when an individual 'malfunctions', it is not that they are 'broken' or 'sick'. It is usually indicative of a much wider problem, or problems, in our social systems that we need to name and start to tackle.

Being a forensic psychologist can sometimes feel like roller-skating on a slippery path. The core challenge is to balance the rights and needs of the client while also satisfying the rights and expectations of my other, indirect clients – you, the public – who, quite understandably, expect to be kept safe from harm. The 'mad' and 'bad' stereotypes conspire to make it very difficult for me and my colleagues to satisfy both camps (and that is without the added pressure of being shouted at in a text message in the wee small hours of the morning).

Our perceptions matter. They impact our politicians' populist, yet ineffective, policies, packing our prisons to the rafters. They impact the way in which 'dangerous' psychiatric patients and 'evil' offenders are funnelled down narrow 'correction' pathways that sometimes support them but more often fail them. And they impact the person who struggles in silence with their own mental distress, too ashamed or afraid to seek help.

I believe it helps to share as much as I possibly can about my job with the society I serve. I hope that you've been able to see my clients as I strive to – realistically, but always with a degree of hope, humanity and good humour. I understand that it's not always easy. It can feel daunting to find yourself in a place of moral ambiguity, where the possible answers to questions of who and what is responsible come in conflicting shades of grey. I wouldn't be at all surprised if there have been moments when you've wanted to turn back to more solid ground, because who wouldn't want to tread a path unpitted by uncertainty? A path where all the signposts are clearly written in black and white.

But life is not like that.

It takes commitment to abandon the 'mad/bad' dichotomy in favour of the far more messy and conflicting reality. In the public conversation about mental health, alongside the celebrities encouraging us to talk more openly about our emotional states, I want to hear more everyday stories about the group with the least-listened-to voices – people who struggle with the most severe and debilitating forms of mental disruption. Only then can we better understand their experiences and where they stem from and counteract the toxic drip of misinformation about the dangerousness of such distress.

We need the introduction of a new professional and public language for the newsworthy occasions when things do go wrong. One that pulls all the different threads of a person's experience together. Encompassing compassion and accountability, it needs to name what each individual is going through, or has gone through, alongside their behaviour. Whether we are in a court-room, hospital ward or perhaps writing a magazine article or documentary script, we must stop reducing people to diagnostic stickers and one-word descriptors and endeavour instead to explain but not excuse, contextualize but not absolve.

If we want to find a collective way forward in addressing the reasons for people's emotional distress, and the unwanted behaviours that sometimes accompany it, we must first learn to tell new and better stories.

ENDNOTES

Chapter 1   The Bright Line

032   *For starters, the vast majority*   Craissati, J, 'Severe mental illness and violence: Understanding risk and responsibility for those who are violent', in Craissati, J, *Forensic Case Histories: Understanding Serious Offending Behaviour in Men*, 2021, pp.106–124

033   *In 2010, Professor Allen Frances*   Greenberg, G, 'Inside the battle to define mental illness', *Wired*, 27 December 2010, available at www.wired.com/2010/12/ff-dsmv/ (accessed 15 May 2021)

033   *one quintillion symptom*   Allsopp, K, Read, J, Corcoran, R and Kinderman, P, 'Heterogeneity in psychiatric diagnostic classification', *Psychiatry Research*, September 2019, no.279, pp.15–22

045   *Dr Kevin Dutton, research fellow*   Dutton, K and McNab, A, *The Good Psychopath's Guide To Success: How to Use Your Inner Psychopath to Get the Most Out of Life*, 2014

052   *In* They Say You're Crazy   Caplan, P J, *They Say You're Crazy: How the World's Most Powerful Psychiatrists Decide Who's Normal*, 1995

Chapter 2   Do No Harm

062   *In* The Memory Illusion   Shaw, J, *The Memory Illusion: Remembering, Forgetting, and the Science of False Memory*, 2016, p.xii

083   *Over time, this fucking thing*   Fisher, C, *Shockaholic*, 2011

083   *What is the sense of*   Hotchner, A, *Papa Hemingway: A Personal Memoir*, 2004

083 *I'm convinced that*   Read, J., 'Why are we still using electroconvulsive therapy?', BBC News website, www.bbc.com/news/health-23414888, 24 July 2013 (accessed 15 May 2021)

084 *Read went on to conduct*   Read, J., Kirsch, I. and Mcgrath, L., 'Electroconvulsive Therapy for Depression: A Review of the Quality of ECT vs Sham ECT Trials and Meta-analyses', *Ethical Human Psychology and Psychiatry*, 2019, vol.21, no.2, pp.64–103

Chapter 3   In Lies, Truth

095 *Office for National Statistics (ONS) data show*   Broadhurst, K, Alrouh, B,Yeend, B, Harwin, H, Shaw, M, Pilling, M, Mason, C and Kershaw, S, 'Connecting Events in Time to Identify a Hidden Population: Birth Mothers and their Children in Recurrent Care Proceedings in England', *The British Journal of Social Work*, 2015, vol.45, no.8, pp.2241–60

102 *By playing sick, we*   Feldman, M D and Yates, G P, *Dying to Be Ill: True Stories of Medical Deception*, 2018

105 *Like the famous Baron*   Asher, R, 'Munchausen's Syndrome', *The Lancet*, 1951, vol.257, no.6650, pp.339–341

106 *He noted that both*   Meadow, R, 'What is, and is not, "Munchausen Syndrome By Proxy"?', *Archives of Disease in Childhood*, 1995, vol.72, no.6, pp.534–8

107 *Professor Meadow's opinion was*   Allitt, Re. England & Wales High Court (Queen's Bench Division), 6 Dec 2007, available at www.casemine.com/judgement/uk/5a8ff77160d03e7f57eac7d7

108 *His erroneous claim that*   'Royal Statistical Society concerned by issues raised in Sally Clark case', press release issued by the Royal Statistical Society, 23 October 2001, archived from the original PDF on 7 April

2008 and available at https://web.archive.org/web/20080407224224/
http://www.rss.org.uk/PDF/RSS%20Statement%20regarding%20
statistical%20issues%20in%20the%20Sally%20Clark%20case,%20
October%2023rd%202001.pdf (accessed 15 May 2021)

117 *She was already one* 'The data', *Pause: Creating Space for Change*,
available at www.pause.org.uk/why-pause/the-data/ (accessed
15 May 2021)

118 *It is 95 per cent women* Robins, P M, & Sesan, R, 'Munchausen
Syndrome by Proxy: Another Women's Disorder?', *Professional
Psychology: Research and Practice*, 1991, vol.22, no.4, pp.285–90

119 *in 2019, women and girls* Taylor, J, 'How do mental health
services blame women?', in Taylor, J, *Why Women Are Blamed For
Everything*, 2020, pp.201–14

120 *Studies have shown that* Timoclea, R and Taylor, J, *'Demonic Little
Mini-skirted Machiavelli': Expert Conceptualisations of Complex Post-
Traumatic Stress Disorder (CPTSD) and Borderline Personality Disorder
in Female Forensic Populations*, 2020

120 *Studies have shown that* Johnstone, L, *Beyond Diagnosis and Disorder*,
2017, available at www.adisorder4everyone.com/downloads-2/

Chapter 4   A Frank Confession

138 *Scott Bonn, professor of* Bonn, S, *Why We Love Serial Killers: The
curious appeal of the world's most savage murderers*, 2014, p.4

147 *Bergwall was originally sent* Day, E, 'Thomas Quick: The Swedish
serial killer who never was', *The Observer*, 20 October 2012,
available at www.theguardian.com/world/2012/oct/20/thomas-
quick-bergwall-sweden-murder (accessed 15 May 2021)

149 *Harrison's downfall came* Perrie, R, 'Yorkshire Ripper Peter Sutcliffe

brands "phoney" serial killer "expert" a liar over £15k speeches about him despite "never meeting"', *The Sun*, 10 July 2019, available at www.thesun.co.uk/news/9481661/peter-sutcliffe-serial-killer-expert-liar-wazzock/ (accessed 15 May 2021)

155 *A 2019 YouGov survey* 'Men have more relaxed attitudes to sexual abuse of boys by women like Emmerdale's Maya', *Barnardos.org.uk*, 4 March 2019, available at www.barnardos.org.uk/news/men-have-more-relaxed-attitudes-sexual-abuse-boys-women-emmerdales-maya (accessed 15 May 2021)

Chapter 5   Snap Decisions

169 *It was her fault* 'Man Accused of Killing Wife in Dispute Over Mustard', *AP News*, 9 July 1987, available at https://apnews.com/article/d11d294fddd5139dad32f68512bce7be (accessed 15 May 2021)

172 *The crucial difference being* Coroners and Justice Act , c. 25, Part 2 Chapter 1, Partial defence to murder: loss of control, 2009, available at https://www.legislation.gov.uk/ukpga/2009/25/part/2/chapter/1/crossheading/partial-defence-to-murder-loss-of-control (accessed 15 May 2021)

177 *As the 2020 Femicide Census highlighted* Long, J, Harvey, H, Wertans, E, Allen, R, Harper, K, Elliott, K, Brennan, K, with Ingala-Smith, K and O'Callaghan, C, *Femicide Census Report*, 2020, available at www.femicidecensus.org/wp-content/uploads/2020/11/Femicide-Census-10-year-report.pdf (accessed 15 May 2021)

180 *The Femicide Census data show* ibid

192 *The Femicide Census found* ibid

193 *In her book* Monckton-Smith, J, *In Control: Dangerous relationships and how they end in murder*, 2021

Chapter 6 An Empty Room

200 *the way in which his body* Sentencing remarks of Mr Justice Spencer in The Queen -v- Joanne Christine Dennehy, Gary John Stretch, Leslie Paul Layton and Robert James Moore, 28 February 2014, available at www.judiciary.uk/wp-content/uploads/JCO/ Documents/Judgments/the-queen-v-dennehy-sentencing- remarks-28022014.pdf (accessed 15 May 2021)

200 *I know it sounds selfish* Laville, S, 'Tetra Pak heir Hans Kristian Rausing admits preventing wife's burial', *The Guardian*, 1 August 2012, available at www.theguardian.com/uk/2012/aug/01/tetra- pak-rausing-pleads-guilty# (accessed 15 May 2021)

213 *You lose her in pieces* Irving, J, *A Prayer For Owen Meany*, 1989

221 *George Bonanno, professor of clinical psychology* Bonnano, G A, Wortman, C B, Lehman, D R, Tweed, R G, Haring, M, Sonnega, J, Carr, D and Nesse, R M, 'Resilience to loss and chronic grief: A prospective study from preloss to 18 months postloss', *Journal of Personality and Social Psychology*, November 2002, vol.83, no.5, pp.1150–64

222 *More than mere tools* Jarrett, C, 'The psychology of stuff and things', *The Psychologist*, 26, August 2013, pp.560-65

222 *But trend forecaster* Wallman, J, *Stuffocation: Living more with less,* 2015

Chapter 7 Pork and Prejudice

232 *John Dovidio, a professor* 'Understanding your racial biases', *Speaking of Psychology*, American Psychological Association, November 2015, episode 31, available at www.apa.org/research/action/speaking-of- psychology/understanding-biases (accessed 15 May 2021)

256 *Surveys of adolescents receiving* Funk, R R, McDermeit, M, Godley, S H and Adams, L, 'Maltreatment Issues by Level of Adolescent Substance Abuse Treatment: The Extent of the Problem at Intake and Relationship to Early Outcomes', *Child Maltreatment*, no.8, pp.36–45

260 *an invisible package of unearned assets* McIntosh, P, 'White Privilege: Unpacking the Invisible Knapsack', *Peace and Freedom*, July/August 1989, available at https://psychology.umbc.edu/files/2016/10/White-Privilege_McIntosh-1989.pdf (accessed 15 May 2021)

Chapter 8 Out of the Hot Seat

269 *Currently, the prosecution of* Centre For Women's Justice, End Violence Against Women Coalition, Imkaan and Rape Crisis England & Wales, *The Decriminalisation of Rape: Why the justice system is failing rape survivors and what needs to change*, November 2020, available at www.endviolenceagainstwomen.org.uk/wp-content/uploads/C-Decriminalisation-of-Rape-Report-CWJ-EVAW-IMKAAN-RCEW-NOV-2020.pdf: (accessed 15 May 2021)

269 *Dominic Willmott, a researcher* 'Researcher calls for "judge-only" rape trials to combat jury bias', University of Huddersfield website, September 2018, available at www.hud.ac.uk/news/2018/september/rape-case-jury-bias/ (accessed 16 May 2021)

270 *Psychologist Jessica Eaton* Eaton, J, 'Women: How to be the perfect victim of sexual violence', *victimfocusblog.com*, 3 February 2019, available at https://victimfocusblog.com/2019/02/03/women-how-to-be-the-perfect-victim-of-sexual-violence/ (accessed 16 May 2021)

271 *In years to come, however* Mews, A, Di Bella, L and Purver, M, 'Impact evaluation of the prison-based Core Sex Offender

Treatment Programme', *www.gov.uk*, 30 June 2017, available at https://www.gov.uk/government/publications/impact-evaluation-of-the-prison-based-core-sex-offender-treatment-programme (accessed 3 April 2021)

274 *The first sign of 'compassion fatigue'* Figley, C R, 'Compassion fatigue: Toward a new understanding of the costs of caring', in B H Stamm (ed.), *Secondary traumatic stress: Self-care issues for clinicians, researchers, and educators*, 1995, pp.3–28

279 *Social worker Malcolm Holt collected* Holt, M G, 'Elder Sexual Abuse in Britain: Preliminary Findings', *Journal of Elder Abuse and Neglect*, 1993, vol.5, no.2, pp.64–71

279 *Another rare study found* Ball, H N and Fowler, D, 'Sexual offending against older female victims: An empirical study of the prevalence and characteristics of recorded offences in a semi-rural English county', *Journal of Forensic Psychiatry and Psychology*, 2008, vol.19, no.1, pp.14–32

292 *Former prison psychologist* Forde, R A, *Bad Psychology: How forensic psychology left science behind*, 2018, pp.111–19

294 *who are three times more likely* 'Child sexual abuse in England and Wales: year ending March 2019', Office for National Statistics, 2020, accessed online at www.ons.gov.uk/peoplepopulationandcommunity/crimeandjustice/articles/childsexualabuseinenglandandwales/yearendingmarch2019#characteristics-of-victims-of-child-sexual-abuse

294 *Approximately 1 per cent* Craissati, J, 'Understanding how sexual victimisation in childhood might be linked to the abuse of others in adulthood', in Craissati, J, *Forensic Case Histories: Understanding serious offending behaviour in men*, 2021, pp.106–24

Chapter 9   Blood, Sweat and Fears

318   *Not only that, but research shows*   Silva, E, 'The HCR-20 and violence risk assessment – will a peak of inflated expectations turn to a trough of disillusionment?', *BJPsych Bulletin*, 2020, vol.44, no.6, pp.269–71

334   *As Professor of Psychiatry Joel Gold*   Gold, J and Gold, I, *Suspicious Minds: How culture shapes madness*, 2014

338   *Those with serious mental*   Brekke, J S, Prindle, C, Bae, S W and Long, J D, 'Risks for individuals with schizophrenia who are living in the community', *Psychiatric Services*, 2001, no.52, pp.1358–66

340   *Psychotherapist and activist*   Watson, J, 'There's an intruder in our house! Counselling, psychotherapy and the biomedical model of emotional distress', in Watson, J (ed.), *Drop The Disorder: Challenging the culture of psychiatric diagnosis*, 2019, pp. 223–36

READING GROUP QUESTIONS

In the Prologue, the author says of the people in the book that 'there may be a little bit of their story in all of us'. What character or moment most resonated with you and why?

In Chapter 1, what factors do you think swayed the jury in Michael's case? Was justice served? What, in your opinion, would be the ideal outcome in this story?

Evelyn (Chapter 6) was not diagnosed with 'hoarding disorder' because it hadn't yet been added to the *DSM* (which the author calls *The Big Book of Human Suffering*). Do you think that this diagnosis would have helped her, or not?

Isaaq (Chapter 7) was first convicted of drug-related crimes at the age of 14. Was he a 'delinquent' or unfairly criminalized? Was youth custody appropriate or helpful? Could his path have been changed and, if so, how?

In Chapter 9, the author says that she has 'rejected the notion that there is a separate group of people who are "mentally ill". There are just some who encounter more extreme distress than others as we all try our best to survive what life has thrown at us.' What are your thoughts on this?

At what points in the book did the author experience conflict between her personal feelings and her role as a psychologist? How well did she manage this? Did any of her patients cause you to feel conflicted? In what way? Did your feelings resolve by the end of the story, or remain ambivalent?

Has *What Lies Buried* made you question portrayals of mental distress in 'true crime', fiction or the news? If so, how?

What can be learned from the book and/or improved upon to lessen the discrimination faced by people who encounter mental-health difficulties?

AUTHOR'S ACKNOWLEDGEMENTS

This book would not have come into being but for my editor Claudia Connal's faith in me – thank you. Similarly, thank you to all the readers of *The Dark Side of the Mind*, who took the stories and messages to their hearts and went on social media, left reviews and told other people about the book. I don't want to sound mushy, but the response has genuinely swelled my heart. I'm incredibly grateful to each and every one of you.

What Lies Buried was written under the shadow of a pandemic, and I'm incredibly fortunate that I had a job to do, typing with one finger at my dining-room table, as my former hospital colleagues and other keyworkers kept the UK running. My appreciation to them, to Jonathan Conway at the Jonathan Conway Literary Agency and to my wonderful agent Sylvia Tidy-Harris at Tidy Management. Sylvia says that many beautiful things are created on dining-room tables, so I hope this book is one of them.

Special thanks to Rachel Murphy for your patience, professionalism and general pizzazz. Also to Daniel Coleman-Cooke for casting your expert eye over the earlier chapters. Further thanks are owed to Susan Bradley for your wise counsel, unwavering support and reflexology balls. I'm glad that we got through this process with only one shocked Beaker meme. I must be improving.

Once again, I am indebted to the expertise of the brilliant team at Octopus Books, including Alex Stetter and Karen Baker. Thank you for trusting me, putting up with me and turning this into an actual real-life book that once again I am proud to send out into the wild carrying the Endeavour logo.

As ever, thank you to Kate in the café for the extra Flakes, encouragement and often very loud cheerleading. To my Mum, for the tea and dog-sitting when I was grumpy and wailing, 'I'm trying to write a book here.' And to my dogs, Humphrey and Captain Fur Potato, for mum-sitting and always making me smile.

ABOUT THE AUTHOR

Kerry Daynes is a registered Consultant Forensic Psychologist with twenty-five years of frontline experience. She has often acted as a trusted advisor to the British government regarding the safe management of high-risk individuals and as a psychological specialist in major police investigations. She is the go-to expert the TV networks turn to for commentary and a patron of the National Centre for Domestic Violence and Talking2Minds. Highly respected in her field, she is 'The Profiler' in the award-nominated TV series *Faking It: Tears of a Crime* (Discovery). Kerry's first book, *The Dark Side of the Mind,* received widespread praise.

Follow Kerry on Twitter @KerryDaynes